The Spattered White Coat

Edmund Messina MD

Patients mentioned in telling the stories in *The Spattered White Coat* are depicted in a manner which does not violate their privacy or reveal their identity in any way.

This work is dedicated to the *Bossy Nurse From 6-Main Reese* and all the fine nurses and colleagues depicted in this book.

TABLE OF CONTENTS

ACKNOWLEDGEMENTS

The author appreciates the input and recollections of Jayne Bailey Messina RN, Steven B. Feinstein MD, Connie Castellani MD and Stuart W. Rosenbush MD. I appreciate the fine copy editing and sound advice of Julianne Renee Geiger.

INTRODUCTION

I wrote this book for the general public to read, although medical people may also find it interesting, if not nostalgic. Many physicians have a similar story. This one is mine.

People always wonder about why a person wants to be a doctor. Why go through all the physical and emotional abuse, long hours, and in recent years, the constant conflict with insurance companies and unworthy administrators? The answer is that medicine—specifically Neurology—makes me happy.

This book tells about the beginning of my journey and about the emotional and harrowing experiences that made me into a doctor. This book relates my experiences as a medical student and intern in some of the best and most intense urban hospitals in the country.

These brief vignettes will reflect the wonderment of a medical student and the frustration of interns and residents. It goes through formative events in the large inner-city hospitals where I trained in the wards, operating rooms, intensive care units, and emergency rooms where I spent so much time.

This book is not a novel or a historical textbook. It is not a biography. Instead, it is a chronological collection of strikingly dramatic true events and experiences that molded me as a physician. It is about the events that happen and the way they changed a young doctor.

This book is not for the squeamish, because the practice of medicine is not for the squeamish. Certain events and behaviors in this book may be quite disturbing for some. At times, I may appear very blunt in my choice of words, and in the stories I have chosen to show you. My intentions are not to titillate or sensationalize, but simply to show the events that altered me forever. It is impossible to accurately judge our behaviors unless you have experienced what we have experienced.

The title of this book, *The Spattered White Coat*, symbolizes the grittiness of the setting. We often got splashed with Betadine (a type of iodine) solution when doing procedures or starting IV lines.

I have related these events to the best of my recollection, so please excuse my extrapolation of dialogue and some of the names. I used fictitious names unless otherwise stated. In some ways, this book is the *Who's Who* of medicine. I took artistic license in the telling of these stories, but the stories are all 100% real.

A doctor's training can take many paths. I chose the grittiest clinical rotations and the most intense training programs to prepare me for my career.

My story starts in the mid-1970s when city hospitals and county hospitals were shocking compared to today's standards. The most prestigious academic training programs incorporated rotations in such facilities where medical students, interns, and residents had a tremendous amount of responsibility and supervision only when we asked for it.

Our teams were worked day and night, sometimes to the point of insanity, as I will show you. The pressures were high, the work was hard, and the learning experience was irreplaceable. We worked hard to treat advanced disease and life-threatening situations. We tried to overcome almost impossible odds, fighting against bureaucracy, budgets, and an often self-defeating patient population.

I had the honor and the privilege of learning from well-known and incredibly gifted clinicians and teachers, as well as brave and suffering patients. I have nothing but respect for these people. Please do not interpret my stories as being intentionally dramatic. What you will read is truly the way things were, as I remember them. I offer no opinions, apologies, or excuses. You will read my impressions of these events as they happened and how I learned from them.

I hope reading about these experiences will in some way change you as well. It is hard to understand what goes on in the mind of a doctor, but perhaps this will give you some insight. Perhaps you will then understand how these experiences cannot leave a person unchanged.

Edmund Messina M.D., FAHS

PROLOGUE

My wife, Jayne and I exited Chicago's Dan Ryan Expressway and headed east on 31st Street. Anyone familiar with the South Side of Chicago knows that this is not a great idea, even in daylight.

We were on a nostalgic quest to see something we loved that had died. It was a sad passing and it happened gradually. We needed to say our farewell.

As we crossed Martin Luther King Drive, we passed the Prairie Shores high-rise apartments where my wife used to live, and we made a left.

We were shocked at what we saw. It was almost all gone... the thing we had loved. Michael Reese Medical Center was no more! Its dozens of pavilions and tall buildings were almost all gone.

We drove along the construction fences that blocked off the ruins of what had once been a famous complex of buildings, some that had been designed by famous architects. In the distance, we saw a partly demolished building surrounded by rubble, its crumbling remainder bravely standing, waiting for the next day's demolition. We couldn't drive any closer, so we pulled the car over next to the fence.

5

Because it was early on a Sunday morning, we figured that most of the hard-working felons were sleeping. The place was deserted, so we started walking toward the fence.

Suddenly, we both jumped as a Chicago Police car pulled up behind us and sadistically whooped its siren. I think the cop enjoyed our startled reaction. She pulled up next to us and looked us up and down.

"You people can't go in there. It's all closed up and it's dangerous. What're you doin' here?"

We tried to explain to her that we used to work at Michael Reese and we were here to pay our final respects. She didn't seem impressed.

Suddenly, her radio went off and she cursed and backed out, yelling to us over her shoulder, "Get out of there. There's nothing to see."

We watched her cruiser screech away onto 31st Street and disappear along with the diminishing sound of her siren.

My wife and I looked at each other and shrugged. The cop was wrong; there was indeed something to see. I bent back a loose part of the fence so Jayne could pass through.

As we walked carefully over bricks and rubble, vivid memories came back to me in a rush.

This crumbled street had once been a busy thoroughfare that went past the various pavilions, now crushed, and past the Baumgarten and Kaplan pavilions.

As I looked east, there was nothing but space, providing me with a view of Lake Michigan. The buildings were gone! Along this street once had walked an endless parade of people dressed in white... nurses, technicians, medical students, interns, and residents. On a nice day, they would all be walking outside. In bad Chicago weather, they walked through the intricate maze of tunnels that connected the many pavilions. At one time, this was the premiere hospital in Chicago, which had always been bustling. Ambulances were constantly screaming into the emergency room and there was an almost endless bustle of cars dropping people off or picking them up at the main entrance in the Kaplan Pavilion.

In my mind, these white uniformed ghosts were walking, as they always will in my memory—medical students trying to keep up with fast walking interns, nurses coming off shifts and laughing—all of them will continue to live inside of me.

To our left was the demolished parking structure that had once been a grassy knoll. I remember how the green grass had once been dotted with couples in white uniforms sitting on borrowed hospital linens, eating picnic lunches for a few stolen moments at midday.

We walked along saying nothing, almost dazed, as we slowly made our way among the ruins. Straight ahead was the partially demolished Main Reese building, built in 1907.

When we got closer to it, my wife became tearful. I just stared as a thousand flashbacks streamed through my head.

The reason for this reverie at the beginning of this book is that this once-great hospital played a large role in the events that brought me to now. Much of my story and my evolution as a doctor started here, during the Golden Age of Michael Reese Hospital.

The following story will tell about the struggle of getting into medical school, getting my internship, and getting my first-choice medical school rotations that I had at Reese. It had been my first choice from the beginning.

Now that you see how this fits in, the story will begin.

PART I
GETTING INTO MEDICAL SCHOOL
THE HARD WAY

HOPE

How the heck could I be too old to get into medical school? I was only 27 years old! Here is what happened...

In the early 1970s, I was working by day as a minor hospital administrator. By night, I was in the graduate program at the Illinois Institute of Technology, heading toward a PhD in molecular biology. I was fascinated by cellular membranes and contractile proteins. As I write this, I realize how dry this probably sounds.

As I went to work each day at the Michael Reese Medical Center on the south side of Chicago, I felt out of place in my civilian clothing, surrounded by tired looking, unshaven, and scraggly looking young doctors in white.

It didn't take long for me to realize that *I needed to be* one of those scraggly looking people with spattered white coats. They looked like they were having a great time, if being physically exhausted and overworked constitutes a great time. I honestly wanted to become one of them. I could sense that they had a strong camaraderie and I was missing it.

Unfortunately for me, in the 1970s, medical schools had an age cutoff policy for freshman medical students. You could not start medical school as a freshman if you were going to be older than 26 years of age at the time of enrollment.

I personally met with the admissions officers at each of the medical schools in Chicago. They all told me pretty much the same story: *I would be too old by the time I became a freshman medical student.* In other words, 27 was just too old!

For some reason, the last school I visited was the University of Illinois College of Medicine on the west side of Chicago. The admissions clerk told me the same thing, but this is where fate stepped in. If you don't believe in destiny, you've never experienced it.

There are a few pivotal moments in each of our lives where a single event bumps our life onto a very different course. Such an event occurred that day at the admissions office at the University of Illinois. After the clerk politely gave me the same bad news as the other schools, a different secretary was standing by the door and motioned me over. I swear that this woman must have been an angel.

"I couldn't help but overhear. The age thing, right?"

I nodded and smiled at her. I probably looked dejected and pathetic.

"Are you in grad school in any of the biological sciences?"

I nodded and wondered what she was driving at. This was interesting.

"There is a special program called the Advanced Placement Examination. Have you heard of it?"

I shook my head. I asked myself, *who was this woman?*

"As part of the University's commitment to producing at least 300 new doctors per year, we need to fill the vacancies from people who drop out during or after their freshman year."

This seemed crazy to me. I asked, "Why would anyone drop out of medical school?"

"Each year, about ten people either decide it is not for them or lose interest altogether. On rare occasion, they fail their courses."

All I could say was, "Wow!"

I couldn't believe it! The University needed to fill every seat!

This angelic person — whose name I never learned — led me down the hallway to another office and introduced me to Dr. Marten Kernis. He asked me to sit down. I was not accustomed to this courtesy, but I quietly sat down. He was not much older than I was.

He explained pleasantly, "The University offers an examination each year that is open to science graduate students, which is basically the freshman final examination."

He asked me about my academic background, and apparently I had enough prerequisite courses from my undergraduate biology degree and graduate school to qualify.

"Are you interested?"

"Yes, I am." I didn't know what else to say. I wondered if I was just having a cruel and highly realistic dream.

Dr. Kernis continued. "About a hundred people have already signed up for the examination. It will be offered about a year from now and we usually have about ten openings to fill."

"How many people did you accept this year?"

"Ten out of about 110 people taking the exam. This year, they were all professors in the basic sciences."

He paused, trying to read me.

"Tell me about your life experiences in the past few years after getting out of college."

As I told my story, somewhat redacted, I wondered if I was hanging myself.

"Wow! You've been a lot of places and done a lot of interesting things...Perhaps a bit scary as well. Do you think you can buckle down and study your brains out for the coming year? There are no guarantees, and you may well be wasting a year of your life. If you're in the top ten and we only have nine openings, you're out of luck. Understood?"

All I could say was, "I can do it." He'd probably heard that one before.

He looked at me for a moment; I could almost see his mind racing and weighing everything. After all, I didn't even have a PhD yet.

He leaned forward onto his desk. "Okay, I'll sponsor you for the exam. I think we need to broaden our usual dry candidate base. We need a little variety."

I stood up and thanked him, shaking his hand. He took a packet of paper from a desk drawer.

"This is the course list for the entire first year program. I can't give you the exact course material, but on the last page is a list of recommended books. You'll need to figure out for yourself what to concentrate on."

I quickly flipped through the pages, and my eyes almost popped out. I think he heard my audible gulp.

He told me that the list looked worse than it really was and that he would be available if I had any questions.

It was surreal. I walked out of the admissions office and onto South Wood Street. I turned around and looked up at the words inscribed above the entrance, "The Abraham Lincoln College of Medicine." I was in shock, and I just wandered around the medical campus with a lightheaded feeling.

I wondered what it would be like to be one of the students who were walking around in short white coats and carrying little black medical bags. I wondered whether I could really learn all the material and somehow pass the freshman final.

The first year of medical school is perhaps the most difficult because it involves the learning of massive volumes of information and a great deal of memorization. The question was whether I could do it on my own... Literally on my own.

My wandering took me a couple of blocks north and I walked through the front door of Cook County Hospital. It was enormous. To me, there was something very inspirational about a large urban charity hospital. The place was teeming with doctors, nurses, and police officers. There were poorly dressed people staggering around aimlessly, people walking with canes, and others being pushed in wheelchairs.

OVERWHELMED

I went across the street to Logan Brothers Medical Books. The store represented my future. On those shelves was my ticket to a new life.

I browsed around the store, looking at the medical instruments in the glass display cases. There were reflex hammers and stethoscopes, and yes, black leather medical bags. White coats were hanging on a clothing rack. The rest of the store was mainly bookshelves and book displays.

I saw medical students and interns browsing through the books. I looked at the book list that Dr.

Kernis had given me. I figured I would begin with human anatomy.

I waited in line to make my purchase, feeling like an outsider in this hallowed shop. I bought my first medical book, *Gray's Anatomy*. It was thick and daunting.

When I got home and opened it, it seemed like there was no way I could learn every drawing from this encyclopedic book of anatomy with countless detailed drawings in tiny print. It was over 1,000 pages. I was overwhelmed.

HOPE AGAIN

The following day, I went back to Logan Brothers and browsed again. I noticed that a girl in the short white coat of a medical student was looking at some books.

I walked over to her and I explained that I was taking the advanced placement exam. She looked at me as if I was a freak. I was dressed in my work clothes. I probably looked like another "suit." She paused a moment and then smiled.

"Use *Gray's* as a reference, not as a textbook."

She led me over to a shelf with other anatomy books. "I used this one last year. It's got all you need for the exam."

She paused. "But wait. What about the lab? Aren't you going to do dissections?"

She was right. I needed access a cadaver as well. I would call Dr. Kernis later.

We talked for a while. She was just about to start a surgical rotation at County across the street. She was buying a pocket-sized light blue book, which was the

Cook County Hospital Intern's Handbook (I can't remember the exact name).

She patted the book. "This is supposed to be all you need to know when you work at County. It's full of formulas and procedures."

We all need books. After she left the store, I kept browsing. I began to feel more hopeful and I bought a couple of anatomy study guides as well.

STUDYING

I had no idea what a medical curriculum would look like or how difficult the tests had been for the medical students. I figured that since the average medical student at the University of Illinois was probably pretty smart, I had better learn everything I possibly could. After all, you run a lot faster when there's a bear chasing you.

From that day onward, I studied night and day. When I felt comfortable with anatomy, I loaded up on physiology books and then I moved to the other disciplines as the months went by. I spent every spare moment studying; every evening, every weekend, and I'm embarrassed to admit, a great deal of my time at work.

Many of you may already know that administrators spend a lot of time in meetings, and I discovered that I could do my job effectively in about two hours per week by avoiding unnecessary meetings and wasted time. Perhaps I am a horrible person, but I don't feel guilty about that.

Part of my lack of guilt was because of my immediate boss at Michael Reese was Ronald Albrecht

MD, Chairman of Anesthesiology. He was very supportive and he encouraged me to give it my best shot.

CRUSHED

About six months into my studying marathon, devouring as much information as I could, I called the admissions office to find out whether the exact date of the examination had been set. The secretary told me that they had changed the rules, and now only full-time graduate students were eligible for the examination.

I was crushed!

I rushed over to the campus and literally ran from my car to the administration building. When I appeared at the reception area, Dr. Kernis's secretary could tell I was troubled. She ushered me into his office. He gave me a warm smile as I explained the situation. He told me he would honor our original agreement.

You see, when I first found out about the examination, I cut back my evening course schedule and was no longer considered a full-time graduate student. I obviously needed the time to study. Dr. Kernis told me not to worry. I thanked him about ten times, and I rushed out the door to go home and study. At age 27, I knew that I was fighting for my life. If I was going to make my dreams come true, this was my shot.

Crazy as it sounds; I had the image of the Michael Reese interns burned in my mind. My dream was to become one of them.

Dr. Kernis also arranged for me to go into the anatomy lab with the other students, if I wished. I wished! I went over there as often as I could, and they allowed me in the lab certain evenings of the week.

EXAMINATION DAY

The second half of my preparation year went by too quickly; I was convinced that I had not studied enough, although I had been through every freshman textbook and every study guide that they carried at Logan Brothers and in the Student Bookstore.

The examination was to be given in the basement of the College of Pharmacy, located across the street from the original University Hospital. I nervously went downstairs to the exam room and gave my name to the proctor, along with the eligibility letter, which Dr. Kernis had sent me. I already knew that I would be one of the few examinees who did not already have a PhD. I was surrounded by professors in the basic sciences who wished to enhance their careers by getting an MD degree. I was up against a bunch of professors! That definitely didn't do wonders for my morale.

The test was to last eight hours per day for two days, and it would consist of all the final examinations that the freshman medical students needed to pass in order to enter their second year. I chose a seat toward the back, took a deep breath, and began answering questions, being careful not to make any stray marks. I'm generally pretty good at taking tests, and they usually don't make me very nervous, but this was The Big One. This would change my life forever, and everything I had was at stake.

About halfway through the first morning session, I was keeping up pretty well, and I was somewhat confident about my answers. Then the anatomy section started. It was *neuroanatomy*, and at the time, it struck fear into me.

In the midst of this anxiety, I happened to slide my test paper off to one side and I noticed that some genius had carved something into the wooden surface of the beat up old desk. It said SUZAN SUX. Somehow, it struck me funny and I struggled to stifle a laugh. It broke the stress and I was able to complete the rest of the exam that morning without too much trepidation. I still chuckle about poor Suzan.

During the lunch break, I started talking with the pretty, red-haired girl, Marianne, who had sat next to me in the exam. She already had a PhD in Microbiology and seemed very bright. We had lunch together, and tried not to say, "What did you get on number seven?"

We told some jokes, which helped to bring down our stress levels. I liked her.

The afternoon session seemed to go pretty well. That is, until the final hour when the questions came back to brain slice anatomy.

The brain is a complex organ and contains many three-dimensional features, which are almost impossible to visualize unless you cut the brain into slices and reconstruct them in your mind. The idea is to remember, from slice to slice, the way a structure is shaped and located so that you have a three-dimensional concept in your mind. I felt like I was struggling through it. When the time was up for the afternoon session, I put down my pencil looked around.

As people were standing and stretching, I was quite convinced that I had wasted an entire year of my life. I was surrounded by people with far more education than my simple BA and partly completed PhD. They looked very confident, if not smug, and that didn't help.

Marianne must have been watching my facial expressions because she came up to me.

"So, what do you think?"

The way I looked at her gave her my answer. I felt defeated.

"Ed, this was a pretty difficult exam. I doubt anyone feels confident. I sure don't."

I smiled at her attempt to make me feel better. "I don't see any point coming back tomorrow..."

Marianne grabbed my arm. She had a surprisingly strong grip. I'll never forget what she said.

"You're an idiot if you don't come back to finish the test tomorrow."

She meant it. Another angel.

I did come back the next day, and sat with Marianne. We both took the rest of the examination. At the end of that day, I was relieved that it was over, but I was convinced that I needed to be realistic and forget about ever getting into medical school. I was in a funk and it was not going to lift for a long time.

GOOD NEWS

About two weeks later, I arrived home after a boring day at work. I opened my mailbox and found a letter from the University of Illinois College of Medicine. It was a thin envelope and I figured that it contained a single-page rejection letter. My heart was doing megaflops. I ripped it open and frantically read it. There were actually two pages; the first page was a letter signed by the Dean, Gerald M. Cerchio MD.

The letter said that I was one of the 10 people selected for admission to the second year of medical studies at the Abraham Lincoln School of Medicine at the University of Illinois. They called the admission "advanced placement" and I needed merely to fill out the second page and enclose a check for $25 to hold my spot open.

I honestly thought that someone was pranking me. The first thing the following morning, I called the Dean's office from my office phone. The secretary chuckled and put him on. For some crazy reason Dr. Cerchio was standing right there. He chuckled and told me that indeed, there was no mistake. He suggested that I go and have a drink.

School was to begin in three months. He congratulated me and said that more than a hundred people had taken the exam and that I had done very well. I imagine that the professors who took the exam had less of a feeling of urgency than I did. I was the desperate one and I guess it paid off. Again, you always run faster when you feel the threat.

As soon as I hung up the phone, I rushed from my office to tell Dr. Albrecht the good news. He shook my hand, and I could see that he was genuinely happy for me, while putting in a plug for me to consider the specialty of Anesthesiology.

As of that time, it was the happiest day of my life. Within a few weeks, I received paperwork for the James Scholar program. It was an independent study program and I was eligible because the Dean had recommended me.

Needless to say, even though I wasn't sure what it was, I signed up for it. I was assigned an advisor, Dr. Mabel Ross from the School of Public Health, a national figure. Well before school started, Dr. Ross invited me to her beautiful apartment on Lake Shore Drive, along with another student she was advising named Dave, also a James Scholar. She was a great advisor, and she helped me a great deal throughout medical school.

On those first days, I felt like an outsider at the medical school. I was older than the other students, and didn't share the bonding of the first year with my new colleagues.

Dr. Ross, bless her heart, sponsored me to take additional examinations that allowed me to quiz out of the didactic courses for the first half of the second-year program, including Pathology and Pharmacology. She also sponsored me to take Part 1 of the National Board Examination ahead of schedule.

Perhaps it was Dr. Ross's gentle method of encouragement, but I again hit the books — very hard — to successfully get through those examinations. Actually, I worked my ass off. School was about to start, and I was going to begin directly in the clinics. No classrooms or lectures. I actually had credit for one and a half years of medical school before I even started.

First lesson learned: It pays to work hard.

...And that's where the adventure truly begins.

PART II
MEDICAL SCHOOL AT THE
UNIVERSITY OF ILLINOIS

DAY ONE

One of the most memorable moments of a physician's life is the first day of medical school. I didn't know what to expect since, until that moment, I hadn't taken the same path as the other students.

Since I had quizzed out of all the lecture classes, my first day of medical school began in the clinics. I was quite excited, but I had no idea what to expect, except that I was going to learn how to take a medical history and perform a physical examination.

This meant that I needed equipment. I had heard rumors that the pharmaceutical companies gave money into a fund that distributed a black bag, ophthalmoscope, and stethoscope to every second-year medical student. I went to the student bookstore to check it out.

It turned out that last year, my classmates opted out of any gifts from outside commercial interests. That meant that I needed to scratch up some money to buy some equipment.

I must say, it was exciting to possess actual medical tools. I bought the equipment that was on the list posted in the bookstore, and I carried it in my little black bag. Very cool.

The first step in my clinical training began with learning the art of physical diagnosis. Physical diagnosis, or "P-dog," is where we learn how to properly ask questions of a patient and examine them. It sounds a lot easier than it actually is. I had no idea what to expect.

History taking, which is the systematic interrogation or questioning of a patient, is a fine art. All the right questions need to be asked, and the art is knowing how to ask them to get clear answers. There are thousands of possible questions that could be asked of a patient. The idea is to be thorough without getting bogged down in unnecessary detail.

You need to lead the patient into telling you things, but you need to guide them into giving you relevant information. This is where the errors of omission will lead to the wrong diagnosis. As a physician gains experience and knowledge, the questions become more efficient. A skilled physician can take a detailed history in a fraction of the time it takes a medical student to do the same history without missing anything of importance. This takes years of experience.

Social skills are important when asking intimate and potentially embarrassing questions, and you need to politely interrupt and guide the patient into telling you what you need to know. A good history is not a simple checklist of questions and answers. The most skilled clinicians can ask leading questions and let the patient just start talking and then guide the direction of the conversation. When done properly, the patient doesn't even feel like they are being interrogated.

The patient's responses to some questions can lead to more questions, so you need to know the significance of the patient's responses. Sometimes the questions are linear and sometimes they are branching. Sometimes a combination of answers will just click, setting off additional questions.

On top of this, as if this was not difficult enough, doctors need to observe the subtleties of body language to see whether the patient is telling the truth or being evasive. It is critical to see how the patient looks at their parent or spouse when certain questions are asked.

Just as the history involves talking and observing, the physical examination involves touching and observing. It is the systematic examination of the whole patient, including their skin, eyes, nervous system, heart, lungs, abdomen, and all the rest. The idea is to look for any abnormalities that can support or refute what was found in the history.

Simple observation tells us a lot about a patient, such as how they are dressed; whether there are tattoos or scars or needle tracks, how worn one shoe is compared to the other, whether there are nicotine stains on their fingers, etcetera. It's all important.

A well performed history and physical is still the most important diagnostic tool we have. Unfortunately, the lack of these skills is the greatest weakness in today's medical system. Perhaps because I'm a neurologist — where history and physical are critical — I think it's important that we improve on the way we teach these skills to new doctors, although greed will always cause some doctors to shorten the face time with their patients.

Getting off my soapbox and jumping back to my early days, I had not yet started learning those skills. I was like an empty container, waiting to be filled. I was a useless medical fixture at the time, but I was enthusiastic... and I had tools!

PHYSICAL DIAGNOSIS - FIRST ATTEMPT

Dr. Ross had arranged for me to begin formal training in physical diagnosis at Cook County Hospital.

"County," as we called it, was at one time considered one of the world's premier teaching hospitals since World War II. Many innovations came from County Hospital including the world's first blood bank and the surgical fixation of fractures. At one time, it had grown to over 3,000 beds.

When I was a medical student there, County was experiencing a certain amount of decay from bad politicians and low budgets, but it was still a wonderful clinical facility to learn in. I couldn't wait to get started.

Although I didn't realize it at the time, I may as well have had a sign on me that said "newbie." I had the clean, white short jacket that was typical of a medical student, neatly pressed, and a cheap but stylish tie, clean shirt, and slacks. Needless to say, I looked extremely out of place when I walked between the dirty, large fluted columns at the main entrance, carrying my brand-new black leather medical bag. I still chuckle when I think about how green I must've looked.

It also didn't help that I didn't exactly know where I was going. County is a huge place, its buildings taking up a large city block with its tall dirty-white brick pavilions. I was wandering somewhat aimlessly with a piece of paper in my hand through the main hospital building. On that piece of paper was written a certain room number. The main lobby was crowded with wheelchairs, crying babies, and angry looking young men from local neighborhoods. I eventually found someone who looked like they might give me a straight answer.

She was an Indian doctor wearing a crumpled white coat over crumpled surgical scrubs. She looked down at my white piece of paper, smiled, and told me to go to the other side of the vast complex. She said I should go outside and around the building because it would be faster.

I was already late by the time I got around the huge building and into the unmarked side door. A small conference room matched the room number on my paper. I quietly entered the room and gingerly closed the door behind me, sitting on a chair at the back of the room. I could see that my friend Dave was sitting nearby.

The instructor was a pudgy middle-aged general practitioner, without a white coat or a tie. He had just started introducing himself to the class, which consisted of about 20 students. This was my first exposure to a medical instructor and I was not impressed. Perhaps I had a different impression of doctors, especially professors of medicine, and I was quite unimpressed by the absence of discipline in what he was saying.

He was holding up different instruments, giving them informal names rather than the official terms.

He held up an otoscope and said, "This is what we call an ear thing."

There was a slight titter of laughter, and he continued. He started making jokes about patients, and frankly, I was very disappointed. He was sloppy and I knew that I didn't want to be like him.

After a few more minutes of disappointment, I got up and left the room. I was uncertain what I should do, but this was not where I belonged. As I was leaving, I noticed that Dave was doing the same.

"What the hell was that in there?" Dave asked, angrily.

I shrugged. "I think we need to go back and see Dr. Ross."

We hoofed it back to the School of Public Health. Luckily, Dr. Ross was in her office. She listened to us patiently and then motioned for us to sit down while she turned to one side to make a phone call. After a few moments, she hung up and turned back around, smiling at both of us.

"Good news. Dr. Tom Lad, Chief Resident for the Department of Medicine at the VA, is willing to tutor you two in physical diagnosis for twelve weeks. He's a very good clinician and I know you'll like him."

The University of Illinois Medical School was located within blocks of many hospitals, including the University of Illinois Hospital, the Westside VA Hospital (now called the Jesse Brown VA), Cook County Hospital, and Rush Medical Center, in addition to the Illinois state psychiatric facility and others. To this day, it may well be one of the most populated medical centers in the country.

LEARNING PHYSICAL DIAGNOSIS AT THE VA

Dave and I hurried over to the West Side VA and found Tom Lad going through charts on one of the medicine floors. He was an informal guy with a pony tail and Buffalo Bill facial hair. (It was the '70s, after all.) He told us to call him Tom. He was smart as hell and a great teacher, and he was very patient with us neophytcs. Years later, he became the Chairman of Hematology and Oncology at Cook County Hospital, which added to his other academic honors over the years.

The young Tom Lad told us he would assign us specific readings about individual patients each day, so we would systematically learn how to ask questions about each organ system and learn how to examine these veterans. As Chief Resident, he knew exactly who was "in the house" and what was wrong with them, because he took Morning Report each morning. Morning Report was where the on-call service would tell about all the patients they admitted in the past 24 hours, and the group then reviewed all of the patients in the house and provided brief updates.

It was a dream come true. We had a personal tutor at a hospital full of patients with all sorts of illnesses!

Tom assigned each of us a patient every morning, in keeping with our readings, and at the end of each day we would discuss them and visit our patients together.

Our job was to take a detailed medical history from each patient, which at first took about four hours (the poor patient). Then we would go eat lunch and go back to spend a few hours stumbling through a physical examination and then spend another couple of hours hand writing a long report describing all of our findings.

A medical history is a comprehensive description of the patient's chief complaint, past medical history, and a detailed set of questions about any possible symptoms they might otherwise be having. This is called a "review of systems," which involved questions about each organ system such as the nervous system, heart, GI tract, etcetera. I still insist that there are no shortcuts, and this often can reveal symptoms that the patient didn't think were important enough to mention on their own. There is no short cut. This is human life.

Looking back on those days, I have to chuckle at how slow I was in the beginning. Over the weeks, I got somewhat faster and more confident. Tom was a very patient instructor and never tried to intimidate or demean us. This was not the case for other students who later related their experiences with other instructors.

To give you an example about how much faster a doctor gets over time, by the time I was an Internal Medicine Intern a few years later, I was able to take a thorough history and do a complete examination on eight patients on a busy night. We did not dictate in those days, so you can imagine how awful those long, quickly scribbled notes looked. It would probably take an archeologist to decipher those hieroglyphics.

On the first day at the VA, Tom had us observe him as he did a thorough abdominal examination on a couple of inpatients with "normal" exams. Then he sent us home to read about the examination of the abdomen. There was a lot to read that night, learning about how to palpate a liver, percuss the belly if there was a fluid accumulation, feel for an enlarged spleen, etcetera. I practiced on a girl I knew. She wasn't a medical student... don't ask.

The next day, we met Tom in the cafeteria after he got out of Morning Report. It was a long session. Several residents each supervised a couple of interns who in turn supervised a couple of medical students. Such was the hierarchy. Tom would be aware of all patients. He was responsible for the wellbeing of all the patients as well as the teaching of the service. He was answerable to the attending who oversaw the service.

Tom assigned us a couple of men with liver disease, which was not hard to find at the VA. In those days, most of the inpatients were former World War II or Korean War vets, usually alcoholic and often with advanced liver failure. War does awful things to people, and it contributed in no small way to their psychiatric and substance abuse problems. We had a few young vets from Vietnam, often with drug problems. I had a special regard for those guys and I still do. Call it survivor's guilt.

Tom assigned me a nice man in his 50s who was a chronic alcoholic. He was a former Marine and he had SEMPER FI tattooed on his left arm. His right arm had a long ugly shrapnel scar and there was a lot of muscle missing. He had been in the Pacific. I don't recall his name, so I'll call him Sam. Sam patiently answered my questions as I madly scribbled notes. From time to time, I would apologize for how long I was taking and he would just laugh and say, "I have nowhere to go, anyway."

The problem was I think he was serious.

Many of the VA patients were brought in by the cops when they found them drunk in doorways. On cold days, the paddy wagon would pick up these men and ask if they were veterans. If they were, they dumped them at the VA. The admitting house officer could always find something wrong with them so they could be admitted. Many of them were truly homeless, and Chicago had some brutal winters. I must say, the Chicago cops had a humane streak in them, especially when the wind was so cold that it literally hurt. If the unfortunate souls were not vets, the cops would try to find ways to arrest them so they could spend the night in a warm cell and get a meal. It was better than freezing to death.

When I finally finished my write-up on Sam-the-Marine in the style that might appear in a patient's chart, I met up with Tom and went to the ward. The VA was set up with multiple bed wards, somewhat like barracks. My patient was not in his bed! Tom told me to look in the restroom.

The restrooms at the VA were large, open areas with urinals and stalls, considerably larger than most public restrooms because of all the wheelchairs. The one for this particular ward was a few steps away, and it was packed with guys in wheelchairs, smoking like mad. One man was actually smoking through his tracheostomy, which is a surgical opening in the front of his throat. I imagined he already had throat cancer.

Sam was leaning on the sink, smoking. The VA had a PX, which sold cigarettes for about 7 cents per pack, which brainlessly added to the problem. Government logic.

I waved to Sam and he smiled, stubbed out his cigarette, and put it into a wall receptacle. He hobbled over to me and it struck me that I had forgotten to have him walk during my examination. I don't think I ever forgot again, after suffering the embarrassment of telling Tom a few minutes later when I presented the man's case.

Tom, Dave, and I stood at the bedside as I demonstrated Sam's enlarged liver, which was several fingerbreadths below his ribs on the right side. Tom went on to demonstrate the other features of Sam's alcoholic liver disease, which I had apparently missed. He showed us the small broken capillaries on Sam's face and the yellowish sclera of his eyes. To my embarrassment, he showed us how the poor man had alcoholic cerebellar disease by having him walk for us. This staggering is called ataxia. Tom was very nice about it, but this was still a great example of learning by embarrassment.

Dave and I later remarked that in our entire time at the VA, we never had palpated a normal liver. It wasn't funny.

Lesson learned: Be sure to get the patient to walk when doing a physical.

THE EYE

I was sitting in the cafeteria quietly reading and eating a tuna sandwich when a fourth-year medical student named Harvey sat next to me. He was a braggy sort of guy who believed that he was of a much higher station in life because he was a fourth-year student and I was only a second-year student. I had already had the displeasure of having lunch with him on the previous day.

I'm certain that he must have been a wimp in high school, and he took delight in trying to dominate others. Other than his annoying personality, he also belonged to the most annoying group of people in medical school, namely the fourth-year medical students. Fourth-year students have a little bit of knowledge and a lot of ego.

Fourth-year students were on consultation services for the most part, as electives. This meant that they would walk around smugly with the specialty service and review the work that the poor intern had done in the middle of the night. A fourth-year student has enough free time to read in great detail about any illness, and look like a genius in front of the attending. The poor intern, on the other hand, is too busy trying to keep people alive and doesn't have a chance to read anything before rounds.

Harvey was on a rheumatology consultation service that went around to the different floors and evaluated people with arthritis or other autoimmune illnesses. Rheumatology is an academic Internal Medicine specialty that requires very detailed history and physical taking. Every little detail is important, and a busy intern who is admitting seven or eight people on a night of call doesn't get the chance to see every detail.

I looked up and nodded as Harvey sat across from me. His air of superiority was present in full force.

"How is physical diagnosis going?" he said condescendingly. At a different place and time in my life, I probably would've inserted his tuna fish sandwich up his nose. Instead, I just smiled.

He continued, "We had some really good attending rounds this morning. The intern missed the obvious findings of psoriatic arthritis."

I smiled and kept looking down at my food. He kicked it up a notch.

"You know what that is, don't you? You know, when the psoriasis makes its way across the fingernail. Have you ever seen that?"

I shook my head. He continued. "I felt bad for that poor intern this morning; he totally missed it on his general examination last night."

Just as he was saying this, the poor intern called Harry came up to the table.

He nodded to me and I said hi.

I had talked to Harry a few times in the past. I found him to be knowledgeable and a very pleasant guy. He was a little bit older than the other interns, probably about my age. He didn't try to pull rank on students.

He looked coldly over at Harvey and said, "How is the rheumatology consulting service doing?" Even I, not very good at picking up subtleties, could feel the deserved sarcasm. Harvey missed it.

"It's a very good service. I'm seeing lots of fascinomas."

I could see Harry visibly wince at that word. I later learned that the term "fascinoma" was a disrespectful word for patients who had unusual or obscure illnesses. This word is a favorite of people who are miscreants with personality disorders. The term combines the word "fascinating" with the suffix "-oma" which would connote a type of tumor. The patient didn't have to have cancer to qualify for this degrading name.

Harvey prattled on as Harry and I tried to finish our sandwiches. He was a true piece of work.

Harry suddenly stood up and said, "Harvey, since you are on the rheum service, are you familiar with inflammatory eye problems?"

Harvey lit up, saying, "As a matter of fact, I just reviewed the literature on iritis."

Harry briefly glanced at me as he said to Harvey, "We got a new admit last night which you haven't seen yet. I think he might have some type of inflammation of the iris. Would you like to see him?"

Harvey got to his feet, saying importantly, "Let me take a look. If it's worthwhile, maybe you could ask for a formal consult from our service."

Harvey turned to me, saying, "Have you ever *seen* a case of iritis?"

Harry watched my reaction and stepped in before I had a chance to actually smack Harvey, saying, "Ed, why don't you come with us, this might be very interesting."

The elevators at the VA were almost impossible to catch during lunchtime, so we ran up the three flights of stairs. Harry motioned for us to wait a moment while he went to the bed and spoke to the patient for a moment. The patient was a very thin, older man with a few days worth of white stubble on his face. He nodded as Harry talked to him. He then lit up and smiled, getting a conspiratory glint in his eye, and I could see him nod. Harry waved us over.

Harvey walked confidently up to the bed and didn't even introduce himself. He simply told the man, "I'm going to look in your eyes, okay?"

Harry and I looked at each other while Harvey took out his ophthalmoscope, shined it in both the man's eyes and then started to look in each eye with the scope. He spent a little more time on the left side than he did on the right. He looked up at us and said, "Oh yeah, both sides." The old man looked at him with a puzzled expression.

"Both sides, do you think it's really both sides? Harry queried him. "Isn't that a little unusual?"

Harvey took on his consultant air, saying, "Well, that's what the textbooks will say, but I've certainly seen cases in the literature where bilateral iritis was described."

Harvey then went on to expound upon the other illnesses such as sarcoidosis, inflammatory bowel disease, and other problems when Harry interrupted him.

"Let's let Ed examine the man before we talk about it."

Harvey rolled his eyes, as if anything I would observe would be of no consequence. I reminded myself that we were no longer in Jersey. Harvey would be safe, for now.

I walked over to the right side of the bed and introduced myself to the gentleman. I shined my light in both eyes, noting that his right pupil reacted but his left pupil didn't. I looked into his right eye and I could see no abnormalities of the blood vessels, retina, or the optic nerve.

I walked over to the other side of the bed, remembering that I had just learned that the difference between a lazy doctor and a good doctor is that a good doctor will walk around to the other side of the bed to see the left eye better.

I tried to see into that left eye and I saw nothing. At first, I thought my ophthalmoscope was broken, but I could easily see the light when I shined it on my hand. I just couldn't see into that eye.

I turned to Harry and said, "I can't see in there." Harvey rolled his eyes and made a low contemptuous sound.

Harry turned to the patient, saying, "Okay Mr. Sobel, show us your eye."

The old man reached up and removed his left eye. It was a glass eye! It was no wonder that the pupil didn't react, and it was no wonder that I couldn't see into the eye! Almost on cue, Harry and I looked over to Harvey.

He was busted!

He looked at his watch and said, "I'm late for attending rounds, gotta go." He scurried away.

Mr. Sobel was in on the joke from the beginning. The three of us laughed, but then I got a sobering thought: *What if some doctors actually faked their examinations?* What if a doctor's own ego interfered with the ability to truthfully and accurately evaluate a patient?

Lesson learned: Stick to your guns when you find something on examination, no matter how much it doesn't make sense.

Another lesson learned: Don't fake your physical findings; it's bound to catch up with you.

BAD BLOOD

The next morning after Morning Report, Tom said he had a very special patient for me and he wanted me to be especially careful. That's all he would say, aside from giving me a name and ward number. I could tell from his tone that something was fishy... but what?

I went up to the floor and found Tyrone in his bed. He was 36 years old and a veteran of the peacetime

Army. By now, I thought I was getting pretty crafty. I noticed that he didn't have tracks on his arms, and he actually looked younger than his stated age. He told me that he had never been a drinker or smoker, but that he was always sick. His record showed that he had had a medical discharge from the U.S. Army for various vague reasons.

He told me about how he had chest pain, shortness of breath, blood in his stools, blood in his urine, joint pain, and headaches. At times, he would just pass out.

I continued to ask Tyrone the usual general review of systems questions and he said yes to everything I asked him. He told me that he thought he had "the bad blood," and he didn't think the tests were accurate. He pointed to the urinal on his bedside table, and I could see that the urine was bloody. I had no idea what "bad blood" was, until one of the nurses later explained to me that in parts of Chicago, it meant syphilis. Interesting.

I took careful notes of everything he told me, and then I examined him. Granted, I wasn't exactly an experienced clinician yet, but I really couldn't find anything wrong in his examination. I even did a rectal exam and didn't find any blood. Because Tom had warned me that this was not an easy case, I re-examined him, except for the rectal, and asked him some of the questions over again. It didn't make any sense.

In medicine, we try to find a common thread to seemingly unrelated symptoms and findings. This is sometimes called Occam's Razor, where the simplest hypothesis is often the best. In other words, the hypothesis with the least number of assumptions is often the best.

Tyrone's symptoms just did not fit into a pattern unless he had about fifty different lethal diseases. I was stumped. It was hard grouping his sheer number of symptoms into any rational pattern.

Later that day, when I was presenting his case, Tom started chuckling.

"This man has Munchausen syndrome," Tom explained. "He needs to be sick. If you look at his full VA record, which consists of piles of paper charts, you can see that he is a hospital hopper. Tyrone goes from place to place, hospital to hospital (all within the VA system, I might add, so it is of no cost to him). He always has dramatic symptoms that seem to require hospital admission. This is a psychiatric illness, and what makes it dangerous is that he may also have medical problems.

"The lesson here is the old saying, 'Even paranoids have enemies.' Whenever you're faced with a frequent flyer such as Tyrone, you still need to give him the benefit of the doubt. It is impossible to know if he is crying wolf or not each time."

"So, what about the blood in the urine?"

"Certainly, we'll need to check it out, but I'll bet you dollars to donuts that he stuck himself with a pin and dripped some blood into his urine. We'll get an orderly to observe him pissing into a fresh container and send it to the lab."

Tom's wise counsel was well taken. I have never forgotten this lesson, as you will see later in my writing. For the sake of the record, Munchausen syndrome comes from Baron von Munchausen who apparently was famous for his fantastic and impossible stories about himself.

Lesson learned: It's hard to tell real disease from fake disease, but always give the patient the benefit of the doubt, within reason. If you're suspicious that they are faking, don't do dangerous tests.

SO, YOU KNOW ME?

One day I was asked to go see a man on the ward who was waiting to be placed in a VA nursing home. The purpose of the exercise was for me to observe anything out of the ordinary on this man. I was not supposed to look in his chart.

When I got to his bed, the man was lying there comfortably, looking at a book. He was a very skinny and pale middle-aged white man with a disproportionately protruding belly. He looked up, saw me, and smiled excitedly as if he knew me.

"You're back! So glad to see you! Have a seat." He pointed to a chair next to his bed.

I sat down, saying, "So, you know me?"

"Of course I do, Doc," he smiled broadly.

"Where do you know me from?"

"You know, from the cafeteria."

I thought about it. He probably had seen me down there with the other students. I began to take his history.

"How long have you been here in the VA?"

"I don't know; maybe about a month."

"Do you have any pain?"

"Oh yeah, mainly in my belly."

I continued my questioning, and he had a good answer for everything I asked. He was bright and alert and his speech was clear. This was going to be easy, I figured.

On my general examination, I noticed many small broken blood vessels on his nose, and his liver was huge. I figured he probably had been a chronic drinker.

I got him up to walk and he staggered somewhat. I asked him how long he had been having trouble walking, and he told me that it had just been a few days.

I continued my examination, thanked him for his time, and went back to the nursing station to write my note.

After lunch that day, I met Tom Lad on the floor. He had me present the patient to him, including the history and my examination findings. I told him that the man had been here a month, complained about abdominal pain, and worked as a salesman in an appliance store. He had a wife and three children who were not visiting today, and I continued my entire story. I wondered why Tom was trying to hide a smile.

I described my examination, including his walking; I made a point not to forget mentioning that. Tom held up his hand and said, "Let's go talk to him."

As we approached the bedside, the man recognized Tom and smiled at him. He didn't seem to recognize me. Tom re-asked many of the questions that I had. The patient gave him different answers. The man said that he was single, worked as a used car salesman, and had just gotten here a couple of days earlier.

It was then that I had realized my error. I did not do a mental status examination because the man seemed so lucid.

Tom asked him, "What year is this?"
"1879. Why?"

"What year is this?"

"1954."

"What year is this?

"1984."

Tom kept asking the same question, getting a different answer each time. He asked him again what he did for a living, and the man said, "I'm a cop, can't you tell?"

We left him sitting on the edge of the bed and we walked away about 30 feet. Tom then had us turn around and walk back to him. He was looking around the ward.

As we came back to the bed, the man lit up again with a smile.

"Hey, my two favorite doctors! Long time no see. Where have you been?"

We said hi and asked some of the same questions. He gave us a completely different set of answers. I was quite puzzled.

We went back out to the lobby area and sat down.

Tom asked me, "So, do you think he's faking?"

I ventured a guess. "Maybe. Maybe he wants to get admitted to a nursing home or a psych unit so he doesn't have to work."

"Well, that's a theory. What's the most striking thing about this man?"

I thought for a moment. "Well, I think it's because he's making things up as he goes."

"Bingo. So, why would he do that?"

I didn't have a good answer.

Tom explained to me that the man had Korsakoff's Syndrome.

Then it rang a bell. I remembered reading about this somewhere. It's due to damage to certain parts of the brain that deal with memory.

Chronic alcoholics are often deficient in thiamine, which is vitamin B1. Because vitamin B1 is essential to energy metabolism in the brain, parts of the brain are damaged when people are deficient, especially if all of a sudden they get loaded with carbohydrates.

I tried to sound at least a little bit intelligent. "So how did he fry his brain?"

"According to the story, he apparently was living in doorways and spent a lot of time either drinking hard booze or throwing up. He was extremely deficient in vitamin B1, and when he went to a rescue mission, they gave him a hearty meal. Unfortunately, they were serving a lot of carbs that day."

I looked puzzled.

"If you are thiamine deficient and you suddenly are given a high carbohydrate load, it basically destroys parts of the thalamus and the mamillary bodies in the brain — the memory areas. That's why we give thiamine to just about everyone who comes into the ER."

So, basically, this man who was waiting for placement had only a few-second memory span and he forgot everything as quickly as he saw it. When people have the inability to store new information, they tend to make up answers to fill in the gaps in their knowledge. This is not intentional, and it is called confabulation.

I went back to the ward later on that day and just watched him from a distance. I noticed that he kept reading the same page repeatedly.

Lesson learned: Don't forget to do a good mental status examination. It's a good idea to ask someone the date. Just because a person looks bright and alert doesn't mean they have a properly functioning brain. This may also be true in politics.

THE ELEVATOR GUY

A few days later, I was eating lunch in the cafeteria with a few of the third- and fourth-year medical students. They thought they were pretty cool as they started getting more confidence in their skills. I just sat there, quietly eating and listening to their banter. They talked about their patients, about how high a white count had gotten. One of them had been to a "code," which is when everyone runs to a cardiac arrest. This particular one occurred in the large bathroom on one of the floors.

Their excitement finally quieted down, and we enjoyed our marvelous VA cafeteria food. Then one of the girls piped up.

"Did you hear about the guy in the elevator?"

"No, what guy in the elevator?"

"Apparently, he was one of those demented guys from upstairs. You know, the guys that have a note pinned on the front of their robe."

He was referring to some of the dementia patients who would get lost around the hospital. It's hard to imagine in a modern hospital how these people were free to roam. The nurses would attach a large paper note with a safety pin on the front of their hospital robe with a name and ward number when they were being taken somewhere, such as to x-ray or physical therapy, so they could be sent back to their ward.

"So what happened to the guy in the elevator?"

"Well, he was in a wheelchair and one of the orderlies was taking him somewhere, maybe x-ray. The problem was, they left him on the elevator."

"So?"

"Well, it turns out that he was there all day long, his Foley bag was leaking urine over the place, and he had pooped himself."

"That would get someone's attention. How could that happen?"

"Dunno. Maybe the orderly was transporting two people and he forgot to go back for the second one. Who knows? You know how some of them are..."

"Nice. Very organized. How did they finally find out that the guy was missing?"

"At the shift change, the nurses were making rounds and they couldn't find him in his bed or in the bathroom."

"I bet the newspapers are gonna go nuts on this one. They love a good scandal."

"Probably. Maybe it'll wake up some honchos around here."

"Yeah, right."

INSENSITIVE TERMINOLOGY

Medical students like to talk among themselves. It's a way of coping with all the pressures of learning and trying not to look like idiots in front of their peers. We tried to learn as much slang and terminology as possible so we wouldn't seem like such neophytes when we were on rounds with the more seasoned house-staff.

Harvey, the jackass senior student whom we met earlier in the book, was trying to impress a pretty girl from my class. Admittedly, we were pretty green, and she figured anything he could tell her would be helpful.

Harvey asked the girl, "Do you know what the O-Sign is?"

She shook her head.

"If you're unconscious and your mouth is open, it's called the O-Sign. If your tongue is hanging out, it's called the Q-Sign, and if a fly lands on your tongue, it's called the Dotted-Q-Sign."

The girl laughed nervously and Harvey grinned. I don't think she was very impressed, because she got up and left the table, taking her tray with her.

We learned other terms from other senior students as well as from the interns and residents, including the habit of calling the brain "the squash." Dementia was known as "squash rot."

A popular novel at the time read by all house staff and medical students was the book called, *House of God* by Samuel Shem. Terminology introduced in that book has become regular speech in the medical world. For example, a GOMER was an undesirable person, an acronym for "Get out of My Emergency Room."

It is still a delightfully irreverent book, which strikes a true chord with medical students and house-staff to this day.

Lesson learned: Patients are people.

SUBJECTIVITY... GETTING EVERY DISEASE

In learning about diseases in medical school, and in seeing them firsthand, you can't help but be suspicious that you may have some or all of these illnesses.

For example, one night an old man was admitted, and as the nurses were assessing him, they noticed that he had body lice. That kind of news spreads quickly in a hospital... quicker than the lice. Cleanliness was not his strong point. He lived in a flophouse somewhere and probably had been demented for some time...and he had bugs.

From a distance, I watched one of my fellow medical students examine him, and when she came back to the desk where I was writing my notes, I noticed that she was scratching her head.

Being my usual irritating self, I asked her, "Are you just thinking hard or did you catch his bugs?"

"Very funny." She kept writing her note, but now she had a very serious expression.

A few minutes later, she walked over to one of the nurses, spoke for a moment, and the two of them went to the supply cabinet to get some Quell shampoo. They stocked it there for good reason.

This is a true medical phenomenon. I too have been in the presence of people who had head or body lice, and seriously, even though you know you didn't catch the parasites, you would feel itchy. It always felt better to take a shower when you could.

On my physical diagnosis rotation, when I was learning about the physical findings of cancer, Tom Lad had me examine various people with enlarged lymph nodes. Certain types of cancer will spread to the lymph nodes, and we sometimes can detect large lymph nodes when we examine a cancer patient. Large lymph nodes can also be due to infections. It's such an important finding that the University of Illinois medical school had special rubber pads in the Clinical Simulations Lab to train us how to detect enlarged lymph nodes. The idea was to train our fingertips.

Like all medical students, I inevitably examined my own neck. I found an enlarged lymph node! It was in my left anterior cervical chain, in the front of my neck on the left. I was convinced that I had leukemia or Hodgkin's disease, but I didn't want to know for sure. Denial is a powerful force among doctors and nurses.

A few years later, when I became an intern at Michael Reese, the enlarged lymph node was still there and it was driving me crazy.

I went up to one of my attendings, Dr. Charlie Shapiro, the penultimate oncologist.

"Dr. Shapiro, can I ask you a favor?"

He nodded for me to go on.

"I think I have an enlarged lymph node in my neck."

I'm sure he had heard this a thousand times from medical students and interns who passed through his service, but he was very polite. I showed him where the node was and he palpated it.

"How long has it been there?"

"I first noticed it about three years ago."

He asked me a few questions and then he smiled, "I really don't think you need to worry about it. You should take a break once in a while and maybe even have a drink when you're not on call."

Decades later, the lymph node is still there. It never changed. Every time I feel it, I think about Dr. Shapiro and how he was so patient with me.

Lesson learned: Don't examine yourself.

FEMALE EXAMINATIONS

The physical examination learning process took many weeks as we covered the entire human body and all of its organ systems. Tom remained a very patient and resourceful teacher. The problem was that all of the patients I saw at the VA were males. There were almost no women in the VA in those days. I needed to learn how to do breast exams and pelvic examinations. Tom always had a plan.

Some of the physical examination classes used well-paid volunteers, often student nurses, who would allow the male and female students to examine them in intimate detail. No one was available at the time, so Tom made other arrangements.

He sent me to the gynecology outpatient clinic at Cook County Hospital. County had a huge outpatient population and the clinic was very busy. One of the senior residents, who I will call Dr. Patel, had agreed to teach me to do breast exams and pelvic examinations. She turned out to be as patient as Tom was.

We were standing outside the curtain surrounding the bed where my first patient awaited us. Dr. Patel explained that most of the women coming to the clinic were pregnant or had venereal diseases. The woman on the other side of the curtain belonged to the latter category.

Dr. Patel went behind the curtain and I could hear her soft, accented voice ask the woman, "Would you mind if a medical student examined you?"

The woman had a booming voice and she said, "No problem, as long as he be young and good lookin'." That broke the tension pretty well, and I almost laughed out loud.

The woman was quite obese and in a good mood — too good of a mood. Unfortunately, she was also shockingly immodest.

By the time I came through the curtains, she had kicked off the sheets that were placed over her for the sake of modesty. I later learned about manic-depressive illness. It was probably her hypersexuality that led to her getting sick and having to come to the clinic in the first place.

Dr. Patel showed me how to lubricate my gloved hand and how to warm the speculum. I realized how useful it was to have a woman teach me how to do a potentially painful and embarrassing procedure on other women.

I don't think I looked like I was shaking, but the overly cheerful patient said, "Don't be shy. Ain't nothin' I ain't put in there."

Dr. Patel and I looked over at each other. She winked at me and then I began my examination under Dr. Patel's kind tutelage.

As I was palpating her cervix, the woman let out a scream. I think I might've jumped off the floor when I heard it. She had pelvic inflammatory disease, probably due to gonorrhea, and she was very tender.

The patient noticed that I was visibly shaken and she said, "Don't you worry 'bout me, Honey, you just take care of business and make me better."

Dr. Patel showed me how to culture her discharge and we completed our examination. The woman thanked me as I was leaving the curtained area.

When we came out from behind the curtains, Dr. Patel gave me a mini-lecture on gonorrhea. You can bet that I really scrubbed my hands after that, latex gloves or not.

Other patients I examined in the coming days were not quite so dramatic. I felt so bad for these women. So many of them were scared, especially the pregnant teenagers who came in with their mothers. In that clinic population, routine gyne exams and pap smears were uncommon. Preventative medicine was not a way of life for them.

Women usually came in when they had symptoms. I remember one woman whose vulva and vagina were literally eaten away by cancer when she finally decided to seek help. The importance of patient education and public education cannot be emphasized enough. I knew that Dr. Patel must have become frustrated after spending several years in that clinic, but she always gently and politely made suggestions to these women. She sincerely tried to teach them the best she could.

The rest of the rotation went smoothly. By the time it was over, I felt comfortable enough to move on to inpatient general medicine. I had no idea what would lie in store for me. Dr. Patel was a good role model.

Lessons learned: It always pays to be gentle and patient.

COOK COUNTY ER

I needed to fill in a few weeks before I started my Medicine rotation at the University Hospital. Maybe it was my ego, but I didn't want to feel like a newbie when I got to the floors. I had never been on a clinical rotation, and I was going to be put in with third-year medical students, myself being a second-year student without any experience at all. I figured that I needed to be in one of the more gritty environments to get some hard-core experience.

Because I was in the James Scholar Program, I could pretty much control my entire schedule as long as I had the blessings of Dr. Ross. She suggested that I spend some time at the Cook County Hospital ER. It turned out to be quite a dramatic introduction to clinical medicine.

There was an understanding that U of I medical students could come in when they felt like it and try to help. Needless to say, the staff was constantly overworked and overwhelmed. It was a good opportunity for me to get some experience and for them to get some free labor, assuming I had something useful to give. I needed to learn some skills.

Other students had said that evenings and nights were the best time because of all the trauma and drama. Therefore, on my first day, I showed up at 6:00 PM sharp, coming through the usual patient entrance.

As I recall it, the ER waiting area was huge; it reminded me of a bus station. Almost every chair was filled with someone crying, holding his or her head, or staring blankly at the ceiling. A raggedy man was vomiting into a nearby trashcan.

I walked up to the desk and told one of the clerks that I was a medical student and I wanted to talk to the doctor in charge. As if she couldn't tell that I was a medical student.

She shrugged and said, "Follow me."

We walked through an electrically activated door into a large room with gurneys everywhere. Some of them were occupied by people with IV lines in their arms and oxygen on their noses. I could see a man sitting on the edge of his gurney with his wrists in handcuffs as a large cop stood next to him, looking bored. The man's right eye was almost swollen shut, and I had a feeling that the cop had something to do with it.

We kept walking through this dramatic scene as nurses hustled from bed to bed.

As we walked, I remarked to the clerk, "The waiting room looks pretty full."

"Nope. There are still a couple of empty chairs. When they all start standing around 'cause they can't get seats, that's when they get mean. It's still early."

In those days, there were rows of intake bays where patients were led and asked to sit on a gurney. The nurses would check vital signs and ask some questions, scribbling on the chart, and then physicians would walk over to the next bay. Off to one side, one of the bays led to a doorway marked DISPENSARY.

People were lined up in front of this doorway. Some were sitting and others were standing, hands or arms wrapped with bloody towels or bandages or holding bloody towels to their heads. This is where people got their stitches, unless they were bad enough to go directly to the trauma area. Some people were holding ice packs on their heads. That's the door where she led me.

When I got inside, there was another large room with many procedure tables, about 10 feet apart. A busy intern was stitching up someone's hand and a nurse was getting a teenager onto another table. The clerk pointed to the nurse, grunted, and then walked away, leaving me to introduce myself.

LEARNING TO STITCH

I gingerly walked over to the nurse, noticing that the teenage boy had his right hand wrapped in a dishtowel that was dripping blood. She saw the student ID badge clipped to my jacket pocket. Then, she saw my crisp white coat, rolled her eyes, and motioned me over to where the intern was working. It was suppertime, so there was only one intern there. I gingerly walked over to where he was just finishing some stitches. His hair was uncombed, he had a two-day beard, and spatters of blood and Betadine decorated his dingy white coat.

He walked over to the teenager, grabbed his good hand, and told him to press on the wound.

"Put some pressure on that and I'll be back in a few minutes."

He turned to me. "You here to help?"

I stammered that I was, and he motioned for me to follow him into the back room. A very tired looking resident was sitting there munching on a submarine sandwich with huge bites. He motioned towards the other half of the sandwich sitting on a piece of wax paper on the desk, offering it to me.

The surgical intern was digging around in his briefcase to find a similar sandwich.

I turned to the resident and said, "No thanks, I just ate."

"So, what year are you?"

"I just started my sophomore year. I've got a few weeks before my medicine rotation starts, so I thought I would come here to see what I could learn."

He chewed pensively, and then said, "Well, you came to the right place. Do you know how to suture?"

I shook my head.

"No problem. Ever hear of 'See one, do one, teach one.'?"

I shook my head again.

He gobbled the last piece of sandwich in his hand, wrapped up the rest in its wax paper, put it into a briefcase and snapped it closed. He pointed to it.

"Fontano's sub. Best in town."

I later learned that he was indeed right. The subs, made at Fontano's Market on Polk Street, not far from the medical center, exemplified one of the finest human accomplishments in the world of sandwiches. It remains one of the few remnants of Chicago's Little Italy.

The resident turned to the intern who was wolfing down his food. "Take your time, Buddy, you need a little break. They'll be waiting for you when you come out."

I followed the resident out to where the teenager's hand was bleeding. The kid looked at both of us nervously. He knew something painful was about to happen. He gripped his bleeding hand more tightly.

In the background, I could see the nurses bringing bleeding people to the other procedure beds. This was going to be an interesting night and, the night was still young.

"Watch carefully," the resident said to me, never actually addressing the patient.

He began to unwrap the hand from the bloody dishtowel. The kid had a nasty laceration across his palm and the blood was welling up as the towel was peeled away. The resident asked the inevitable and predictable medical question, "What the hell happened to you?"

The kid looked at both of us. "I dunno, just cut it... I guess."

"Looks to me like you tried to grab a knife from somebody. Am I right?"

The kid didn't answer. He just looked down at his bleeding hand.

"Well, it looks like you're lucky. I don't think you cut any big arteries. Let's take a look at the tendons..."

With that, he pulled on a pair of sterile gloves, took a pair of forceps from the sterile tray which the nurse had placed next to him, and began to poke around in the wound. The kid yelled.

"What you doin', man!"

The resident glanced up at the kid. "Looking to see whether you cut any important tendons. Just sit back and shut up."

In my rather tumultuous life before medical school, I had seen some amazing and awful things, but I was actually shocked at the way this doctor was talking to the patient. It was my first exposure to an emergency physician, and he just didn't seem very sympathetic. He also looked very tired and probably was getting burned out.

The kid just turned his head away and started to whimper. The resident, who I later learned was actually a surgical resident, cleaned the wound, injected a local anesthetic, and showed me some shiny, almost silver, ribbons in the wound.

"These are the flexor tendons. He got lucky and didn't cut them. All we need to do is clean it up, stitch it up, and wrap it up.

I nodded and watched carefully as he proceeded, explaining each step. When we were finished, the teenager looked at his hand, counted the stitches, and let the nurse wrap it up.

He looked up at the doctor, saying, "Hey, thanks man."

He actually thanked the doctor! He was smiling but I could see where there were tears on his face.

We walked away from the kid and the resident let me assist on two more cases. Then he said, "Now it's time for you to do a few."

I was thrilled and nervous at the same time. Since there were so many people with lacerations, there was no shortage of subjects to stitch.

He asked the nurse about the people lying on the beds, and he came back to me saying, "Let's see you do this one."

The patient was a middle-aged woman who stated that she cut herself while cutting some vegetables. The cut was located on the pad of her index finger.

She explained to us, "It just wouldn't stop bleeding so I thought I'd come in here."

The cut was superficial, and it only required a couple of stitches, the resident told me. This was my big moment!

I pulled on a pair of gloves, size 7 1/2, and I draped her wound.

I turned to her and said, "You're going to be fine, I just need to put a couple of stitches in. First, I'm going to give you a little bit of local anesthetic before I start stitching."

She nodded and patiently waited for me to do my job.

The wound was clean but I irrigated it with saline and peroxide. I clamped the curved needle into the needle holder and pulled the thread through both sides of the wound. I was a little clumsy at making the knot, but I remembered how the resident had done it by twirling the thread around the needle holder.

I must admit, I was a little bit shaky because the lady was watching me do the stitching.

"Say, have you ever done this before?"

I looked at her and smiled, "No, you're the first person I have ever stitched up."

She laughed, saying, "You guys crack me up around here."

I had a feeling she might've been tasting a lot of cooking sherry or gin before she cut herself; she was in a very good mood.

I continued with my stitching and my primitive attempts at knot tying until the resident was satisfied that the stitches were in good position. She only needed two stitches. We cleaned her up, and wrapped the wound. I said to her, "You need to come and get the stitches out."

"When?"

I looked over to my resident who said, "In one week have us or your own doctor take out the stitches. Remember, keep it dry and clean."

A nurse came over to bring her out to the discharge area, and she smiled at me. Maybe some people think it's cute when a medical student stitches his or her first patient. I know I felt very good about it.

The resident looked to the line and saw that we were falling behind.

"Okay, Doctor Kildare. I think you got the idea. We need to put you to work. Just be careful about your knot tying. Tight."

As patients were brought in, he checked their wounds and saved the appropriate ones (meaning the simple ones) for me.

He told me, "You're on your own. If you run into trouble, please come and get me."

By the end of the night, which passed very quickly for me, I felt quite comfortable with placing stitches in simple lacerations. I must say it was a surreal experience, and looking back over all the experience I had since then, I think I did a good job at the time.

Lesson learned: Practice makes perfect.

My weeks in the County emergency room were an intensive precursor to the many days I would spend in emergency rooms in the coming years.

By day, I was reading *Harrison's Internal Medicine*, the standard reference book. If you have ever seen this book, you know that it is massive, written by many hundreds of authors, and needless to say, not exactly light reading.

By day, I would strap the huge book to the back of my bicycle and ride along Lake Michigan until I found a quiet place. I would read chapters that I thought might be helpful in the coming weeks. Actually, I selected specific illnesses, which I thought might be common on the inpatient service. I read about heart disease, diabetes, and other conditions, making copious notes and marking up my copy of the heavy book.

Each evening I would go to the emergency room and spend time with different doctors. When suturing became boring, I decided to follow "Dr. Lin." He had been trained in Internal Medicine in his native China before World War II, and now was a full-time employee of Cook County Hospital. I was watching him evaluate a patient with abdominal pain when suddenly everyone started running toward the trauma area.

THE COWBOYS

Two stretchers arrived at almost the same time, and the Chicago Fire Department paramedics ran them to the trauma area. Doctors and nurses converged on them. Apparently, the paramedics had radioed in that they had two black males, about 30 years of age, with gunshot wounds.

According to the cops, these guys had it out with a pair of .45 caliber semiautomatic pistols, cowboy style. Now, in previous life experiences in faraway and hostile places, I've certainly seen my share of gunshot wounds, especially from the GI issued .45's. Now, I was looking at these gunshot wounds from the other side of the barrel, so to speak, from the medical perspective.

The man in the first stretcher was dead by the time he reached the ER. It was no wonder, since he was shot square in the chest; he didn't stand a chance. People sometimes say that a .45 caliber bullet "goes in like a pea and out like a potato." They're not kidding. It's a very destructive weapon.

The other man still had a pulse, but he had very labored breathing. A bullet had hit him in the upper thigh and blood was pouring out of it in pulses. He was bleeding out in front of our eyes.

I kept out of the way and watched the nurses with shears cut off his clothing in an instant while the doctor intubated him. This is where a tube is placed in the trachea that essentially allows the doctor to breathe for the patient.

One of the more senior doctors was shouting orders and everyone was doing their job. It was a remarkable sight; two interns were placing large bore IVs into each arm, and another one was putting something into his groin on the side without the wound. A surgeon was trying to clamp off the pulsing artery. Nurses were carrying bottles of IV saline and packed red blood cells and hanging them on the IV racks. It was hectic but extremely well organized.

The next time you find yourself suffering from a gunshot wound, be sure you're taken to one of these inner-city hospitals rather than a fancy suburban white bread facility. These people knew what they were doing.

I watched every step of the well-choreographed drama until the patient was wheeled away to the operating room. This whole scene took place in just a few minutes, but it was intense. These people have done this so many times that it was like a well-rehearsed ritual. I was impressed. Years later, I would be one of those doctors for a while, although I didn't know it at the time.

Dr. Lin suggested that I go down to the x-ray department to see what the x-ray films looked like. I needed to get some experience looking at x-ray films. They were actually films in those days; no one knew that digital technology was soon to come. We had never even heard of digital technology at the time. I spent a good deal of my time over the next few days in this department.

When I got down to x-ray, naturally there were no films to review because they were going to be done later, once they had the bleeding stopped. There was a radiology resident on duty, and he started showing me x-rays of previous gunshot wounds that they had treated there.

Bullets are very easy to see on an x-ray because they are dense to the penetrating x-ray beam. Military bullets are encased in copper, the so-called full metal jacket. Civilian bullets were often just made of plain lead, and these had a habit of fragmenting or mushrooming when they hit solid tissue.

The resident showed me many examples of bullets from these so-called "Saturday Night Specials," (meaning junk civilian handguns). I find it ironic that Chicago has always been like Dodge City in the old West, despite fanatic gun control regulations.

Now, back to the gunshot victim. Once the surgeons had stabilized his torn femoral artery — a miracle in itself — they took a portable x-ray in the operating room.

The x-ray was quite impressive. The bullet had actually shattered the upper femur. There was additional bleeding from other parts of the injury, and the surgeons were in there for a long time. The man lived.

Lesson learned: Never get shot.

THE GUY WITH THE SWORD

One day, I was sitting with the radiologist in front of a bank of view boxes. The x-ray view boxes were large white Plexiglas panels with florescent lighting behind them. We were looking at routine chest x-rays.

He was teaching me how to look at a chest x-ray and evaluate heart size and vascular congestion, and spot infections such as pneumonia. We were, of course, sitting in the dark with the x-ray viewing screens in front of us. Once your eyes are accustomed to the dark, the x-rays are much easier to view, especially with all the subtleties of shading on these black-and-white pictures.

Suddenly, the door to the viewing room burst open, blinding us for a moment. It was pushed open by a cop who had his revolver drawn.

"Did a guy with a sword come running through here?"

"A sword?" I managed to ask.

The cop was out of breath. "Well, maybe a machete or something. Did you see him?"

The radiologist managed to say, "N-n-no, we didn't."

The cop nodded and rushed back out of the room, slamming the door behind him. The radiologist and I just looked at each other.

This was the nature of County Hospital; it was never boring. As I look back, I wish I could have spent more time there. What made me choose rotations in other places was because I was looking for a more academic faculty. At the time, my plan was to become an academic physician, specialty to be determined.

Certainly, patients are the best teachers, and there was certainly no shortage at County. What I learned from County, however, was that the best teaching takes place in the most extreme places. Although I was looking for academic teaching, over the years, I managed to get most of it in places such as County.

THE NEUROLOGIST AND THE APPLE

One day in the County ER, while shadowing Dr. Lin, we were evaluating a patient who had trouble walking. Dr. Lin said we needed a neurology consult, so he paged the neurology resident on-call. The patient was an elderly Mexican man who looked very worried when Dr. Lin walked away. He smiled when I told him I would stay with him until the neurologist had completed his evaluation.

While we were waiting, I chatted with the man as best I could, while doing my own rudimentary version of the neurological examination. Needless to say, I had him walk. It didn't look good. It mostly looked like a stagger, and at one point I had to catch him so he wouldn't fall. I was quite familiar with these problems from my time at the VA.

Before long, I could see a tall longhaired hippie with a Fu Manchu mustache enter through the staff entrance. He stopped to talk to one of the nurses who pointed my way. He walked quickly over to where I was standing with the patient on the gurney. He was eating a sandwich (not the good Fontano type), which he probably got from the cafeteria.

Chewing noisily, he said, "So, somebody call for a neuro consult?" He looked at my badge and saw that I was a student. He nodded recognition.

"Tell me about him," he said while thumbing through the paper chart. He put the last bit of the sandwich into his mouth, chewed, and swallowed.

He turned to the man. "Hello sir, I'm a neurology resident and I'm going to help figure out what's wrong with you."

He reached into his white coat pocket, I assumed to take out a mysterious neurological instrument. Instead, he produced an apple.

While eating the apple with his left hand, he pointed to the man with his right hand.

"Sir, please stick your arms out in front of you and turn your palms up."

The man did this with no problem. The resident took another bite out of his apple. I could hear the crunch from where I was standing; it must have been a very fresh apple.

"Okay, now touch your finger to your nose with your right hand and then your left hand."

Chomping on the apple with his left hand, he indicated with his right hand how the patient should hold up his fingers, move his eyes and do other elements of the classical neurologic examination.

By now, he had finished the apple and tossed the core into a nearby wastebasket. He made a thumbs-up with his hand.

"Okay now, Sir, let's get you down off this table and see how you walk."

We both helped the man down and the neurologist watched him walk. He was unsteady.

"Now, come back the other way."

I was walking next to the man, so when he started to fall I was able to catch him. The two of us helped the man back onto the gurney and we had him lie down.

The neurology resident motioned me away from the patient. When we were out of earshot with our backs to him, he said, "I bet he has a cerebellar tumor; this came on too quickly. We're going to need a brain scan."

A year later, the CT scanned would make its debut in Chicago. A few years later the MRI would take its place as the most accurate way of looking at a living brain.

However, that day in the emergency room, the best we had to offer was a brain scan, which was a nuclear medicine test. It was somewhat accurate, but unfortunately, not available at night. The man was admitted and I was later told that he had a big brain tumor in his cerebellum, possibly a metastatic tumor from his lung cancer, which was also diagnosed. I don't know what happened to him after that, but I imagine it wasn't good.

JUST A SIMPLE TRIP TO THE MORGUE

Later that evening, Nancy, one of the regular ER nurses, came up to me and asked for a favor from me. She had been kind and patient with me in recent weeks, so of course I told her yes, although I didn't know what the favor would be.

In those days, nurses wore starched white caps and starched white uniforms and sensible white nursing shoes. When they went outside, they would commonly wear heavy blue wool cloaks. It was a nice touch, and actually, I miss that. The new breed of nurses was training at the same time I was. The world was changing, and I was changing quickly, and mainly for the better.

She gave me an odd look and said, "I need help to bring a body down to the morgue."

At first, I thought this was some sort of initiation or practical joke.

"Yeah, right."

"No, I'm really being serious. It's just a simple trip to the morgue."

"Don't take this wrong, but why do you need me to help you?"

She smiled, saying, "Because of some shenanigans in the past, there is a new rule that all corpses brought down to the morgue must be accompanied by a male and a female."

"What you mean by shenanigans?"

"I mean, we live in a sick world and there have been some strange things happening to some of the bodies heading to the morgue."

"Strange, you mean like.. "

She nodded, bringing many nauseating images to mind. It is a sick world, for sure.

"Come on," she said, "Give me a hand. This might be educational for you. It'll be fun!" She had a way of making everything seems smug. I liked her.

We walked over to one of the bays in which curtains had been pulled around the gurney. I've seen many dead bodies in my time, but not in this setting. The deceased was an old white woman with sparse white hair. She was thin to the point of being almost skeletal. She had no teeth; her dentures had probably been removed after her death, probably in the little bag tied to the side of the gurney with her personal effects. Her skin was yellow and blotchy, and her unseeing eyes were sunken deep into their sockets.

I looked at her poor old hands. They were deformed from many years of painful arthritis, and I could see the impressions on her left ring finger where a wedding ring must have resided for many years. Perhaps it was in that little bag with her personal effects. I couldn't help but wonder if those eyes once had a sparkle as she gazed at her first love. How those crippled hands once held her firstborn...

Nancy broke my corny reverie.

"Help me roll her over so I can place this sheet underneath her."

We rolled her and Nancy expertly wrapped the woman in the sheet. She bundled her up like a mummy.

"Check this out. It's her ticket to eternity."

She was filling out a name and hospital ID number on a toe tag. She tied it to the big toe. So, this is how our days would end, I thought to myself. The toe tag summarized our life in just a few words.

I helped her slide the body onto a wheeled cart.

She looked at me, "Hey, you okay?"

I nodded and she continued, "All you need to do is walk with me as we push this cart through the tunnels to the morgue. Are you scared?"

I was quite sure she was kidding, but I answered defensively, "Of course not! What's there to be afraid of?"

Nancy lifted her hands into claws to mimic the predatory grip of a Hollywood monster and laughed. She started pushing the cart and I followed her.

The old woman had come in by ambulance, DOA. I don't know anything else about her story. The nurse told her supervisor that she was going to the morgue and pointed to me. They both nodded and I smiled stupidly at them.

We went down the elevator into "the tunnel." The city morgue was about a block away from Cook County Hospital, and it was reachable by underground tunnel. Ironically, the morgue was near the famous nurse's residence where eight student nurses had been tortured and murdered in 1966 by a mass murderer called Richard Speck.

Although she was a joker, Nancy was not a big talker, so we walked somberly along at a good pace. One of the large wheels on the gurney didn't touch the floor very well and would spin around at times as we cruised through the tunnel. The tunnel was dark with harsh, bare light bulbs hanging from the ceiling about every 30 feet. Big pipes ran along the ceiling, several of them dripping condensation into small puddles on the concrete floor. The wheels of the gurney ran through some of the puddles and left trails on the floor. If I were to make a horror movie, I would film at least part of it in this tunnel.

As we walked, I looked at the shrouded figure on the cart. She was a very slight woman, so she didn't make much of a silhouette on the patched white sheet in which she was bundled. She reminded me of the mummies I've seen in museums — so old, so small, and so frail.

I didn't know whether there was a bereaved family in the Quiet Room of the ER, where bad news is often given. I don't know whether she was simply dumped there from the nursing home. I only know that she was sadly dead. Her race had been run and she was heading for the morgue.

By the time we wheeled the empty cart back to the ER, it was getting late, so I left the ER to go home. As tired as I was, I had trouble sleeping that night. For some crazy reason, that little trip to the morgue made a big impression on me.

Lesson learned: Live life to the fullest. Remember, in the end, your life will be summarized on a toe tag.

DR. REDDY AND THE LIGHT BULB

On one of my days in the ER, I followed the surgical intern around. We'll call him Dr. Reddy. He was a nice guy, very friendly and understanding of my lack of general surgical knowledge. He explained everything to me whenever he could. He had already been a surgical attending in India, but when he came to the US, he had to start over again; hence, he was a very experienced surgical intern. County had many Indian doctors in those days.

The American medical system has very specific rules. If your medical training was done in a foreign country, except perhaps if was done in Canada, you need to take an equivalency examination. Those who pass the examination must then begin their house-staff training like any other medical school graduate in the US.

Many foreign doctors who were doing house-staff training in the US had already achieved a certain amount of recognition in their home countries. Some of them, for political or other reasons, wanted to move to the US, so they started again through the grueling training process.

Language and culture are sometimes a barrier when trying to understand the typical patient who comes to Cook County Hospital. In the ghetto, a common mispronunciation of the word "vomit" is "vomik." I still chuckle when I look back at Dr. Reddy interrogating a patient who had been throwing up. When she said she was "vomiking," he would repeat it in his accent, and it came out as "womiking." That being said, he was a very good teacher, and I believe he ended up as a professor of surgery somewhere on the East Coast.

Emergency room nurses are delightfully cynical and sarcastic, which is probably why I like them so much. Nothing fazes them; they've seen it all. Repeatedly.

In the back room, Dr. Reddy was explaining to me the proper approach to evaluate someone with an acute abdomen when one of the nurses came back.

"We've got a foreign body in 9," she said, and her rising and falling eyebrows made it clear that this was a doozy.

The patient was a 22-year-old graduate student who was both uncomfortable and embarrassed. The nurse stood behind him, arms folded, trying to suppress a grin.

It turned out that this young man had a low wattage light bulb stuck in his rectum. Now, over the years, everyone in medicine has seen such a dilemma utilizing different objects or under different circumstances; it's still all the same. Although we'll never really know why people put these objects into the part of the body which nature has reserved for storing feces, you can't help but ask.

"I don't know..." The young man said, "I was changing a light bulb and..."

I think mainly the reason medical people ask these questions is to see the variety of answers they might get.

We wheeled him down to x-ray, and sure enough, there was a 10-watt light bulb in his rectum, the metal screw threads pointing toward the exit. It was unbroken. Remember, the 10-watt bulb is not large like the common 60-watt variety, but somehow, it got away from him.

We went back to talk to the patient. Dr. Reddy was truly a gentleman as he spoke to this embarrassed young man, putting him at ease.

"We are going to have to put you out so we can relax the muscles and extract the bulb without breaking it."

The young man agreed, and Dr. Reddy got him prepared for the procedure. The challenge is to not break the object or push it in further.

I went back to the x-ray department to look at the film again, and one of the radiologists recognized me. He saw the film I was looking at and smiled.

He asked, "Got a minute?"

I nodded, and he motioned me into his office.

He pulled a thick folder off one of the shelves.

"This is my teaching folder."

He carried it out to the viewing area and he started putting some films up on the screen.

"This is a collection of films showing the different types of foreign bodies that people put into their body cavities. Especially the rectum."

He appeared to have an enormous x-ray collection of these objects. He showed me pictures of light bulbs, pool balls, pens, shot glasses, vibrators, and even a small mayonnaise jar. As you know, such a jar does not have a tapered end. One could only speculate at how it was inserted.

"So, what do you think?"

All I could say was, "Amazing."

Lesson learned: Never be shocked. There will always be something stranger to come.

I was getting a lot of clinical exposure, but I needed to spend more time reading about internal medicine. I took the final week off from the ER and just read my *Harrison's* day and night. I didn't know what to expect, so I wanted to be ready. I had a bad case of that medical student tendency to read. No one wants to appear like an idiot in front of his or her peers.

THE MEDICINE SERVICE

Internal medicine or just "Medicine" is the discipline that deals with patients eighteen and older, as opposed to pediatrics, which deals with the younger crowd. It is one of the most important rotations in a medical school career because this is where you learn how to make a proper diagnosis and how to keep people alive.

As noted earlier, I learned physical diagnosis from the Medicine Chief Resident at the VA, but this was to be a different rotation. Now, I would learn how to actually diagnose and manage diseases such as diabetes, heart disease, cancer, and many other disorders. I was there to learn a proper discipline and approach to medical problems.

I reported promptly at 7:00 AM to the third floor, north wing, at the old hospital previously known as Illinois Research. During my time there, it was called the University Hospital, the main teaching hospital for the University of Illinois. The university was also affiliated with several other hospitals in Chicago, including the VA and Cook County Hospital. I opted for the rotation at the main hospital so I could get some good raw-knuckles medicine. I was told that it was much more intense than the suburban community hospitals.

When I got there, one of the nurses pointed me to the Resident's Room, which is where the house-staff and the students would gather, smoke, go through charts, and in general, share educational experiences. Indeed, at that time, doctors would smoke on the floor in the hospital. The patients could smoke in rooms where oxygen was not being delivered, and the hospital gift shops used to sell cigarettes. Thankfully, times have changed.

The only other person in the Residents' Room was Hannah, a third-year medical student. I introduced myself and we shook hands.

She looked at me suspiciously. "So, how does a second-year medical student end up on the medicine service?"

She obviously thought it was weird that a second-year student was doing Medicine, so I explained the whole James Scholar thing. She listened patiently to my story, but I could tell she was just being polite.

"So, because I started my clinical rotations early, I'll be able to do more rotations."

It seemed to make sense to her, so she nodded. We were still the only ones in the room.

Although I didn't fully understand Hannah's indifference, I was extremely thankful that I was given the opportunity to start earlier. Thankful is an understatement. I still could not believe that I was actually in medical school!

Hannah was an intense person, like many of the female students in my class. Women were not commonly found in medicine at that time. My medical school class was considered radical because we had an unprecedented 17% female enrollment. Hannah's class, which was the year ahead of me, had even less women, so she was truly a curiosity.

Times have changed. The girls in my class had their hands full with lots of gender abuse. Patients always assumed they were nurses because they were women, just like people mistake male nurses for doctors. My female classmates clearly felt that the older surgical attendings lived up to the designation of Pig.

So, Hannah and I sat, waiting. She told me that she had just come off a difficult general surgery rotation, so how hard could medicine be? I told her that I had no frame of reference with which to compare it.

She looked at me with some disdain, saying, "So... Ed, this is going to be your first clinical rotation?"

"Well, I spent a few weeks in the ER at County. Does that count?"

I saw at least the faintest glimmer of respect. It seems that doctors respect each other more when they have been through harder times. My future was going to be chock-full of much harder times than these.

Suddenly the two interns, I'll call them Steve and Clarence, burst into the room, laughing at was probably an off-color and inappropriate joke. This was highly probable because they instantly stopped laughing when they saw Hannah. In the midst of this, Buster, the resident, walked in.

Buster was a senior resident who drew the short straw, so he was obliged to supervise this service instead of getting a comfortable specialty rotation. He was a big guy, always puffing on a cigarette, and he had a certain warmth that made me feel welcome. He looked the two of us and smiled.

"You two are the only students we'll be getting on this rotation. Sorry, but you're gonna work your asses off." He looked for a reaction from Hannah for his choice of words. She didn't budge.

He pointed to me and looked at my badge. "Ed, you are assigned to Clarence... We already know this is your first rotation." Clarence gave him a dirty look.

"And Hannah, you'll work with Steve." Steve smiled at her and she winced a little from the type of smile he gave her.

Clarence glared at Buster. "Can I speak to you in the hall?"

They went out and closed the door. Hannah shrugged.

"So, you pissed him off already?

"I'm good at that."

Steve laughed. "Sorry, man. I don't know what to tell you." He knew why Clarence was mad, but I didn't.

Buster and Clarence came back and Clarence started angrily running a pick through his fro haircut. Again, this was the '70s. To this day, I don't know what his initial problem with me was. I later gave him reason to be mad at me. As I told Hannah, I'm good at that.

Buster had the floor again, lighting up another Marlboro. Clarence was puffing on a briar pipe. "I'm going to have each team operate autonomously, students answering to interns. The interns will report to me midmorning every day and at the end of each day before we do teaching rounds. Our attending will be none other than Dr. Morton Bogdonoff, the Chairman of Medicine."

It sounded good to me. Hannah was stoic, and Clarence said, "Shit. Are you kidding?"

Dr. Bogdonoff had the reputation of being a very demanding and knowledgeable attending. You didn't cut corners when you worked for him, he was a national figure. Although I didn't realize it at the time, Clarence was intimidated by him. I later figured out why.

Buster smiled and clapped his hands together. "So, we all need to be on our best behavior. Ed, be sure you always are wearing a tie. Right? Now let's get to it."

House-staff tend to be intimidated by their Chairpersons. I had previously met Dr. Bogdonoff when I interviewed for the James Scholar program. I liked him and he didn't seem to hate me.

When we talked about my filmmaking background before graduate school, I'll never forget what he told me. He said that since I came from a world of imagination, I would be particularly suited for original research. Years later, I had the privilege of meeting with him at Cornell when I was applying for my Neurology residency and he actually remembered me.

Clarence pulled Buster aside. It didn't seem to bother him that I could actually hear what he was saying.

"Look Buster, I got too much to do, especially if Bogdonoff is going to be the attending. I don't have time to show a brand-new student how to do scutwork."

Buster paused for a moment and then said, "Okay. I'll give you a break for at least a few days. But you've got to get your act together."

In addition, he walked over to where Hannah and I were standing.

"Hannah, since you've just been on a busy service, I want you to show Ed the ropes. You two can help each other."

If Hannah was disappointed, she was too nice to show it. She was very familiar with the drudgery known as scutwork, having already been on a demanding surgical service. In those days, medical students were a plentiful source of free labor for any tasks needed for patient care.

She smiled at me, "Scutwork is scutwork, no matter which service."

Frankly, I preferred to learn from Hannah in the time-honored tradition, which I just learned, of "see one, do one, teach one." Hannah seemed a hell of a lot more hospitable than Clarence. I expected I'd have some trouble with him over the coming weeks, but I had no idea how bad it would get.

She showed me the supply closet.

"All the floors are arranged in the same way. This is a supply closet. It's full of blood tubes, needles, IV tubing, and any other supplies we're going to need. You save a lot of time when you keep blood tubes and Vacutainer needles in your pockets."

She took a length of latex tubing and threaded it through the buttonhole in my white coat.

"This is your tourniquet. We'll be drawing a lot of blood and starting a lot of IVs, if this rotation is anything like general surgery. We are the beasts of burden... the scut dogs."

Hannah showed me how to follow the colored stripes on the floor for different destinations. These were part of the floor tiles and ran along the right side of the hallways at the University Hospital.

"So," she said, "let's say you want to go to the lab. Believe me, you'll be going to the lab a lot. All you have to do is follow the red stripe in the floor. You know, red is for blood."

"You know, I used to be a lab technician years ago, when I was an undergrad."

She gave me her first real smile. "Really?"

"Oh, yeah. I worked full-time nights, everything from phlebotomy to blood bank, from chemistry to hematology."

"That's great! At least I don't have to show you how to draw blood. Every service needs someone who can hit any vein."

From then on, we developed a good collegial relationship and helped each other out on morning work rounds. We were actually a pretty good team.

Other than being expected to do all the dirty work for my part of the service, I got most of my teaching from Buster rather than from Clarence, who was never around. Buster patiently went over my cases with me. In addition, I would sit with Hannah and Steve when they were going over things. I don't know where the hell Clarence was half the time, and I really didn't care.

Students were expected to know about all the patients on the service, and to be particularly up-to-date on certain individual patients, known as "our patients."

THE MAN WITH THE ULCER

At first, because I was a newbie, Buster assigned me a single patient to start with, pissing off Clarence who had to do more work on a service that was already shorthanded. For the sake of privacy, we will call the patient Mr. Curran.

He was a red-faced Irishman with a good disposition. He was in the hospital because of a bleeding ulcer.

This is an example of where medicine has really taken a turn for the better. In the 1980s, it was discovered that many ulcers are caused by a bacteria called H. Pylori... and it is *curable*!

Unfortunately, the pre-1980s era had to deal with life-threatening ulcers such as the one afflicting Mr. Curran. He was admitted with a severe upper GI bleed. He came in through the ER and directly admitted to Medicine. He almost bled out, it was so bad.

In those days, medical students on service were referred to as Doctor in front of patients. All of a sudden, the green Dr. Messina was in charge of a man with a bleeding ulcer. I was being carefully watched, and the patient was in no real danger... at least not from me.

I spend a lot of time with Mr. Curran, and I got to know his wife as well, since she was usually at his bedside. This was an era when there were no business school graduates forcing people out of the hospital prematurely. We were waiting for Mr. Curran's ulcer to heal, and I was checking his blood and his stool each day. We had an NG tube (nasogastric tube) in his stomach, and all seemed to be going well. He was healing, and his hemoglobin was coming up.

I visited Mr. Curran's room several times per day, and I shared with him and his wife my newly acquired knowledge about his condition. He was a smoker and he liked to drink a bit. Okay, he liked to drink a lot. We talked about his habits at great length; my job was to talk him into not hurting himself with his habits. To his credit, he never got angry when I mentioned the need to stop smoking and drinking.

It's hard to convince a patient to stop smoking when you and the entire medical staff are smokers. I did my best to make him feel guilty whenever he lit up if I was walking past the room.

In the coming months, I figured out that patients were more patient with me because I was a few years older than the other medical students.

Otherwise, the service went well. I looked forward to the attending rounds, and I watched the house-staff wilt under Dr. Bogdonoff's precise questions about each patient on the service. I went out of my way to prepare for these rounds, and he was always patient with me. I think this further infuriated Clarence.

Buster could see how things were going, but who the hell was I, an untested medical student, going up against an intern? Clarence, after all, was a medical school graduate who managed to land a position on the University of Illinois house-staff. I was still not very impressed with his knowledge compared to the other intern, Steve.

THE MONKEY ROOM

One evening after a very long day, we finally finished our work and we were about to turn over our service to the on-call team. Steve, Hannah, and I had finished our work, and Clarence was still down in the emergency room with an admission that came in just before the changing of the guard. I already had my admissions for the day, so Clarence was on his own. Buster told him that we would help him out if he got in over his head.

He volunteered my services specifically, should Clarence need help with the scutwork.

"Meanwhile, the rest of you are invited to come to the Monkey Room. Dinner is on me."

Buster, Steve, Hannah, and I went to the infamous Monkey Room. I wasn't sure exactly what that meant.

About two blocks from the U of I Hospital on Harrison Street, right across the street from County, stood a bar and restaurant known as The Greeks. Honestly, no one probably knows the real name of the restaurant. Rumor has it that three Greek brothers started the restaurant.

The Monkey Room was located in The Greeks. If you walked into the bar itself and went to the right, you would find a huge room containing large numbers of people in white coats sitting at tables and eating. This was the main hangout for medical students and house officers from surrounding hospitals. If paged, you could quickly run from The Greeks to County, University of Illinois Hospital, the VA, or Rush Medical Center.

It was a tradition, and all the nursing stations had the number for The Greeks when they were seeking out house-staff or students. The Monkey Room got its name from the mural on one wall, which depicted giant monkeys and palm trees. It didn't look like a particularly Greek theme, but who were we to question?

Hannah explained to me, "The Monkey Room is where medicine is taught. We went here all the time when I was on the surgical service."

The Monkey Room was like a sacred temple of learning, like in ancient Greece. As we sat around the table waiting for menus, Buster had each of us describe our cases while he and Steve made constructive comments. As I looked around, I saw similar conversations taking place at other tables. There were no HIPAA regulations in those days. In fact, some people at the next table actually had brought charts with them!

Food at The Greeks was also somewhat interesting. One of the featured dishes was spaghetti with chili. As a full-blooded Italian American, I got cold chills when I saw that item on the menu. I didn't feel brave enough to try it on that particular evening, although I had it on subsequent visits. It wasn't really that bad.

We sat, talked, and laughed. We told embarrassing stories about each other and had a good old time. I really felt like I was part of the system... I truly felt like I belonged... Except when I had to deal with Clarence.

Lesson learned: Nothing beats camaraderie.

THE SPINAL TAP AND THE BET

In the midst of our eating and hilarity, the public phone rang in the Monkey Room and someone answered it.

"Anyone here named Messina?"

I took the phone. Clarence had stayed behind to admit the patient in the ER, and now the man was starting to go into the DTs, a result of acute alcohol withdrawal.

Clarence pleasantly said, "Messina, get your ass over here and do a spinal tap."

I left my partially eaten burger on the table. Buster told me he would be back later to check on things. He was well aware of my relationship with Clarence. I still didn't know what I had done to make him so mad.

When I got to my floor, Nurse Kelly asked me, "What size gloves do you wear?"

"7 1/2."

She was carrying a spinal tray into one of the rooms, where I could hear yelling.

It's important to know that Nurse Kelly was legendary. She was beautiful, and did not date medical students or house-staff. It made her aloof and even more desirable to all who fell under her spell. Clarence flirted with her whenever he could. She never seemed impressed.

Clarence suddenly appeared at the nursing station.

Raising his voice, he said, "What the hell took you so long?" His glance flicked over to Nurse Kelly to see her response. She ignored him as she walked by.

I could tell this was not going to be a good night.

"Ever do a spinal tap? You know, a lumbar puncture." He enunciated the words slowly, malignantly.

I ignored his tone and answered, "Yeah, I've seen a few done at County and I've done one so far."

"Okay, Hotshot. Here's your chance to do your second one."

I went into the room where the yelling was coming from. A middle-aged alcoholic was thrashing all over the bed while two orderlies tried to hold him down. Nurse Kelly was bedside setting up the spinal tray. She handed my gloves to me. Clarence was standing on the other side of the bed. Everything was happening pretty fast.

"What're you waiting for, Messina?"

We both looked down at the man who was thrashing and straining against the beefy orderlies.

Nurse Kelly looked somewhat uncomfortable. Clarence walked toward the door. He was apparently not going to help me.

As a neurologist, I have probably done several thousand lumbar punctures over the many years since that night. On that fateful night as a medical student, however, it was the most harrowing tap of my career.

A lumbar puncture is performed by holding the patient on their side, in a fetal position, to spread the dorsal spinous processes of the back. After cleansing the skin with an antiseptic, a long needle is inserted at a proper angle, at a level below where the spinal cord ends. Once the needle passes through the membrane that surrounds the spinal canal, fluid drips out into vials, which are then sent to the lab. The purpose of the test, at least in this situation, would be to rule out meningitis or hemorrhage.

The problem was, the man was a moving target and I was on my own. Clarence was not going to help.

In my mind, I reviewed the exact anatomy and the technique that the ER people had taught me at County. Perhaps I looked too confident, but Clarence was set on making this an uncomfortable experience for me.

I looped a long bed sheet behind the man's legs and his neck, forcing him into a fetal position. I had seen this done successfully in the ER. They called it the Bellevue Sheet Technique. I showed the orderlies how to twist the sheet to keep it in control and I put on my gloves.

The man was thrashing and now he was beginning to have a seizure. He was convulsing, but he still was in a good position to get the needle in. The clock was ticking fast. In a few more seconds, he would be straightening his back out completely. I painted his back with Betadine solution and began to insert my needle.

From behind me, I could hear Clarence trying to impress Nurse Kelly, loud enough so I'd be sure to hear it above the man's shouting.

"Kelly, I bet you five bucks he can't get this tap."

She ignored him and I worked on controlling my anger. The patient was getting worse by the second, and it was crucial that I get the spinal fluid. If Clarence had cared about the patient, he would have been helping me.

I advanced the needle slowly until I felt a pop as my needle passed through the dura, which is the membrane lining the spinal canal. Excellent! I slowly removed the central wire from the bore of the needle, and fluid began to flow. By now, the patient was thrashing wildly, but I was able to collect a couple of ccs of cloudy fluid, obviously infected. As he was beginning to hyperextend his back, I pulled out my needle. Mission accomplished!

When I looked down at the needle, it was bent. I apparently pulled out the needle in just the nick of time.

I turned to look for Clarence, but he was gone. By now, Buster had arrived. Kelly handed him a syringe and he was pushing some IV Valium to stop the seizure. The convulsions slowed down.

Kelly handed him the tube with the spinal fluid in it and he held it to the light.

"Nasty looking fluid. That had to be a difficult tap."

I grinned; the sweat was still on my brow. Kelly smiled at me. Wow!

"Did Clarence help you with this?"

Kelly piped up, "No. Not a bit. He did this by himself."

Lesson learned: Don't let anyone shake you when you have an important job to do. Deal with them later.

Buster had Hannah start a second IV for antibiotics. As suspected, the patient had bacterial meningitis, and we all had to take preventative antibiotics for a few days until the cultures came back.

If any medical students are reading this, DON'T DO WHAT WE DID without looking at a CT or MRI image. Doing a spinal tap when a person has a mass in their head is dangerous. We just got lucky. The thing is, at that time, CT scanning was not yet available. It arrived in Chicago the following year.

THE DEAN'S LETTER

Since we are on the topic of Clarence, let's jump to the future for a moment.

After all these years, I'll never forget Clarence, (again, that is not his real name). In retrospect, I'm quite convinced that he probably was a bad physician. In addition, he certainly wasn't a literary genius, because when he wrote his assessment of my time on his service — my report card — it was a bit of a mess. He gave me an awful evaluation.

Years later, I sat with Dean Cerchio to go over my entire medical school record so that he could construct my Dean's Letter. This document summarized a student's overall medical school performance. It was a key element in the application process for residency.

Dr. Cerchio was a great guy, and the students loved him. We felt that he was fair and a true student advocate.

He looked at my folder, which contained evaluations from all my clinical rotations. He was flipping through the pages.

"Messina, you have a weird record. I was reviewing it before you came in. You have no classroom grades other than the classes you quizzed out of... Nicely done, by the way. My letter of recommendation will be based on the evaluations from all of your clinical instructors."

I didn't know what he was building up to. I was certain that I had only good evaluations since I started.

"You seem to have gotten the most out of the James Scholar Program. Your list of attendings looks like the Who's Who of medicine. They all seemed to think you did an outstanding job... Except for an intern on your first clinical rotation."

Clarence!

He closed the folder.

"When we see an evaluation which deviates so much from the others, including that of your attending and resident from that same rotation, we have to consider that there must have been a personality clash."

I nodded, waiting to see where this was going.

"This intern who didn't like you was not a literary genius. Frankly, the poor grammar and spelling in that evaluation is an embarrassment to the University. Hard to imagine how he got this far..."

I chuckled.

"Needless to say, we will disregard that evaluation."

Dr. Cerchio wrote me a great Dean's Letter, which paved the way to the internship and residency of my choice.

Lesson learned: Do your best, always. It always catches up to you in a good way.

THE BLEED

Within a week of his admission, Mr. Curran seemed to be doing better; his blood count had improved and was holding steady. Buster said that we could discharge him in another couple of days, as long as his hemoglobin remained stable.

I was taking a rare moment to review a chapter from *Harrison's* in the teaching room when I heard screaming.

"Come quickly."

It was Mrs. Curran! I rushed to Mr. Curran's room, and could not believe what I saw.

He was sweating profusely and looking scared to death. He had an emesis basin next to him full of vomited bright red blood and clots. I could smell another strange odor coming from the darkening sheets below him. Nurse Kelly was on the spot. She ushered Mrs. Curran out of the room. At that moment, Mr. Curran's eyes closed, and Kelly rushed over to feel his carotid pulse.

She shouted, "Cardiac arrest. Call a code!"

For a moment, I was frozen to the spot. A split-second later, Buster and Hannah were in the room. Nurse Kelly had jumped onto the bed and was doing chest compressions while another nurse pushed the red crash cart into the room. She was so aggressive with her compressions that her cap had fallen off.

Buster quickly intubated the man, yelling to me, "Here, bag him!"

I grabbed the Ambu bag and started breathing him.

We all worked as a team.

I turned the bag over to the respiratory therapist who had just arrived, and I started a second IV on his other arm while Hannah rushed in with bags of normal saline per Buster's instructions.

She yelled to Buster, "Packed red cells are on the way. Good thing we had four units on hold."

Nurse Kelly pulled back the sheets and we were overwhelmed by the powerful odor of digested blood. Mr. Curran had lost control of his bowels, and there was a black tarry liquid all over the bed between his legs. His unconsciousness spared him the embarrassment. There is no smell like digested blood.

We eventually got him stabilized, and we transferred him to the ICU and then to emergency surgery. The surgeons were able to control the bleeding, and he was transferred to the post-op surgical floor a few days later. He didn't come back to our service during that admission because he then "belonged" to the surgeons.

After he was discharged, he and Mrs. Curran came by our floor to visit. He made a point to thank each of us personally. They brought a box of chocolates for Nurse Kelly. I was beginning to understand why people loved medicine so much. I still do.

JEROME

On a quiet Sunday evening, I was writing my notes for a new admission when Hannah came up to me.

"I've got this heroin addict in Room 7, and I can't get a decent vein. Steve wants me to draw some blood and start an IV before this guy goes into withdrawal. He's got SBE."

SBE stands for subacute bacterial endocarditis, an infection of the lining of the heart. It can be the result of using dirty needles. It is an actual infection of a heart valve that can throw small clots to small blood vessels, like the in brain or in the skin. When it goes to the brain, it can produce a brain abscess. It is very dangerous and can cause severe heart damage.

Hannah was a pretty independent and capable person, but she counted on me to find those impossible veins. It was my gift.

She updated me. "This guy is a real piece of work. You'll see."

When we got to the room, there was a lot of yelling. The patient, who we will call Jerome, was doing the yelling.

Jerome, a 22-year-old from the neighborhood, was a serious heroin user and probably a small-time dealer. He was grabbing his left hand with his right, and Steve was trying to talk him into letting him start an IV. Steve was exasperated. He looked at Hannah and me.

"This gentleman has the symptoms of bacterial endocarditis, probably related to his intravenous heroin use. I've got someone waiting for me in the ER, so I'm leaving him to the two of you. He's got to have an IV stat. If you can't get a line in him, get the surgeons to come over to do a cutdown." He purposely looked at Jerome as he emphatically said the word "cutdown."

Jerome's eyes opened wide. He apparently knew what a cutdown was, having been admitted numerous times to this hospital.

A cutdown is a procedure where an incision is made over one of the deeper veins, usually in the wrist, and a semi-permanent intravenous tube is stitched into place. It's not the most pleasant procedure, but there were not a lot of options at the time.

Steve left the room and Hannah asked me to take a look at Jerome's hand. He had tracks in all the visible veins of his forearms and backs of his hands, except for a small vein near his left index finger.

In those days, heroin was brown and expensive, and it left dark traces in the veins. Because of the frequent use of heroin, most junkies would very precisely place the needle only a couple of millimeters from the previous needle injection site, hoping to get as much use as possible out of their remaining veins.

Jerome was a mess.

I touched his hand and he tried to pull it away as I said, "Jerome. Please let us start the IV. You need this medicine in a bad way." I could feel the heat of his fever under my hand.

We finally settled him down, showing him that we had no needles in our hands.

Hannah said, "Jerome, at least let us look at the vein."

Sure enough, there was a nice robust vein near the left index finger that he was guarding from us. It was one of the dorsal metacarpal veins.

"Jerome, that's a beautiful vein," I said. "I promise I'll be gentle with it."

Jerome grabbed the hand again. "No way, man."

Hannah held up a 22-gauge butterfly needle. This type of needle has wings on either side so it can be taped carefully onto the skin. This type of needle also allows a very low angle of approach, sparing even the smallest vein, if done correctly.

It took about 20 minutes of argument and threats of serious disease before he finally agreed to let us place the little butterfly needle into that precious vein.

I taped his hand firmly onto an IV board so he wouldn't flex or move his hand. He didn't like it, but I think we convinced him with the threat of dying from a heart infection.

Once we had Jerome tucked in, Hannah said, "Listen to his heart."

She could see my eyebrows go up as I listened. She nodded knowingly.

"He's got a murmur," I said.

"Yup."

The murmur made his diagnosis of SBE even more likely, and even more dangerous. I had just been reading about subacute bacterial endocarditis, and I thought I was pretty much a hotshot to catch that murmur.

You get that way when you're a medical student whenever you learn something new. For some reason, you think you're the only person in the world who knows that new fact.

You become especially obnoxious when you become a fourth-year student on the consult services.

You have the luxury of reading about every illness in exquisite detail, and when you go on rounds, the poor bedraggled and exhausted intern hates you. We've seen that one before.

I reached down and picked up Jerome's hand, shining my pocket light on his fingernails. I said, "Splinter hemorrhages."

Hannah picked up his hand and looked at the small streaks of blood under his nails, caused by bits of material thrown from his heart valve into circulation, being trapped in the capillaries under his nails.

She looked at Jerome. "Jerome, I'm going to keep a close watch on you. Believe me, we will do the best we can to help cure this infection."

Jerome did not look impressed. He just nodded and turned away from us.

MIDNIGHT MADNESS

The rest of the evening was quite boring, and it was starting to get late, close to midnight. I had just finished my last note, and Hannah looked like she was in between tasks.

I said, "So, you want to go over to County for some midnight madness?"

She looked up at the clock and said, "Yeah, why not? After all, it's free."

In those days, Cook County Hospital kept one of its dining halls open and loaded a long buffet table with stacks of lunchmeats, bread, and cheese to make sandwiches. It was intended to feed the on-call house-staff since they didn't get a chance to sleep anyway.

Those of us that had been to County on previous rotations knew about this opportunity, which we called midnight madness. We all felt that our free labor at one time or another entitled us to a free meal. It seemed normal for free food to be available to underpaid or unpaid trainees. At least *we* thought so. It was supposed to be a tradition, like when you feed actors and crew on a film set with the Craft Services table.

Hannah and I walked the two blocks over to County. It was in one of the closest buildings so we didn't wear coats. University of Illinois medical students were constantly warned not to carry our black bags at night, and to be sure that we covered our white coats if possible.

Apparently, there was an ongoing threat of muggings. It never made sense to me why anyone would mug a poverty-stricken house officer or medical student. I guess they thought we had drugs or needles on us. Regardless of how nonsensical it was, reports of armed robberies were a reality.

We were walking so fast we were almost out of breath. Hannah said, "I am truly starving."

"Me too."

She looked worried. "What if we get mugged?"

"I'm so hungry that if a mugger came up to me, I'd probably eat him."

When we got there, the main doors to the dining room appeared to be closed. We were wearing our student ID badges in case someone asked, but no one ever asked this late at night.

She looked disappointed. "Shit, I bet we're too early."

I pushed on the big doors and they swung open.

We were early, so none of the other "diners" had arrived yet. We entered the big dining hall, and at the far end was a long table with the sandwich fixins' stacked on it.

When we got to about 20 feet from the table, Hannah froze and let out a scream.

There was a huge brown rat walking across the cold cuts, making his away from the salami to the cheese stacks. It seemed such a shame with all that good food going to waste. We left before anyone else even got there.

When we were back outside, I asked, "Still pretty hungry?"

"Damned right. It takes more than a rat to kill this appetite. I'm starving."

"How about the Monkey Room if it's still open?"

We never went back to enjoy midnight madness again.

Lesson learned: Don't knowingly share food with rats.

LEAVING THE GROUND

It is very common for medical students and residents to fall asleep in conferences. Once the lights go out to show slides or x-rays, about 20 percent of the group begins to nod off. This was not a reflection of the quality of the presentation; it was merely a symptom of the long hours we spent on the wards.

Throughout this account, you will see references to sleep deprived medical students and house officers. Certainly, tragedies have occurred, but not related to patient care. I have had colleagues who were in serious and even fatal automobile accidents because they fell asleep at the wheel coming home from long shifts on call.

One night while on the medicine service, I was coming home from a 36-hour call schedule with almost no sleep at all. I was driving my old Triumph TR-6, a type of English sports car with a very short wheelbase.

I pulled out of the medical center and headed east on the Eisenhower Expressway. It was late, and if I hurried I would be home by 2:00 AM so I could get at least a few hours of sleep and then be back for work rounds at 7:00 AM the next morning.

There was no one on the road, and I was flying down the highway. The last thing I actually remembered was passing under the large post office building, which straddled the highway. My next memory was that of a loud roaring from my engine, and I opened my eyes to see that I was in the air!

I think it was Wabash Avenue that formed the hump at that time. As I hit that hump, I must've become briefly airborne. The rear wheels of my short little car left the ground and the engine spun to about 5,000 RPM. It certainly got my attention because I snapped awake and frantically grabbed the wheel.

Luckily, there was nobody crossing Wabash, and I landed safely. My wheels were probably only a couple of inches off the ground, but it was enough to spin the engine. The whole thing probably only took a few seconds, but I remember it like a slow-motion scene in a movie.

I pulled over to the side of the road for a moment to collect my thoughts and to look around to see if anyone saw me... like a cop, for example. Luckily, the place was deserted so I continued on my journey, considerably more alert. The adrenaline lasted for quite a while, and I didn't really get to sleep like I was hoping to when I got home.

Lesson learned: Don't drive if you're too sleepy.

By the end of my 12-week medicine rotation, I felt quite comfortable about the workings of a hospital service, and I was getting very good at scutwork. Medical students are the cheapest form of labor in a teaching hospital. In fact, they actually pay the University to work for free. It's worth it, even though we had to draw blood, transfer patients, and start IVs and all the other stuff to keep things working.

By now, I was quite familiar with the University of Illinois Hospital. I knew where the labs were, where x-ray and the pharmacy was, and where all the other services were located. I had a good idea of how to make things work for me.

The standard joke in the medicine department was the answer to the question, "How do you treat diabetic ketoacidosis?" The answer was, "Draw a red top, a purple top, and a green top tube, put the green top tube on ice, walk down the hall, go down three flights, make a right and hand it to the lab technician."

As much as we complained about the scutwork, these rotations were making us tough. We became efficient, and we made every step count. These were important skills for when we became interns, and I felt like I could handle most things on a medical service. I would later find out that I had a lot more to learn.

Nevertheless, I didn't feel like a newbie anymore and I was ready to move to my next rotation, which was General Surgery.

GENERAL SURGERY

If the Medicine Service was the Army, then General Surgery was the Marine Corps. There was strict discipline, a very rigid chain of command, and shades of grey did not exist. In surgical logic, the only colors are black and white.

My first surgery rotation was also at the University of Illinois Hospital, but on a different floor. I was assigned to a surgical intern named Cort, and our resident was a red-haired daredevil they called Red. There were two teams on the service, and we took turns with night call. That meant that we were on call every other night!

Surgeons are a funny brood. According to the classical story, a surgical intern was complaining about being on call every other night. The attending's response was, "You're right, it's a shame because you're missing half the cases."

At Illinois, the Internal Medicine doctors were called "fleas" by the surgeons, because they jumped from bed to bed on rounds and lingered before hopping to the next bed. The medicine people called the surgeons "blades" for the obvious reason. It was friendly animosity.

Surgical work rounds were early in the morning so the surgeons could get to the OR for elective surgery.

The team on call could be doing emergency surgery at any time. We had to be around, in house, at all times when on call. No more Monkey Room on on-call nights.

We covered patients both at the University Hospital and at the VA. We often ran back and forth when we were on call.

I loved General Surgery. It was hardcore, intense, and there were no uncertainties. Our attendings were famous surgeons, literally.

At this point, I have to admit that I intentionally manipulated my schedule, thanks to my James Scholar status, so I could select the clinical services run by the Big Guys at U of I, the VA, County, Rush, and Michael Reese hospitals. I figured that I might as well be taught by the people who literally wrote the book. I was extremely lucky to have that opportunity.

In keeping with that thought, our supervising attendings, Dr. Robert Baker and Dr. Lloyd Nyhus, were the editors of the *Manual of Surgical Therapeutics*, the house-staff bible. I always had a copy of the book in my pocket. When I was on Medicine, I had the *Washington Manual of Medical Therapeutics* in my pocket. These clever spiral books were made to fit in the pockets of white coats and have been invaluable for trainees since the 1940s. Now, of course, they exist in our smart phones.

I had picked a tough service. The surgical residency program was structured like a pyramid. A starting resident had no guarantee that he would be allowed to enter the next year. There was a lot of competition among the residents, who tried to outdo each other for the sake of survival.

The University of Illinois Hospital, in addition to Cook County Hospital, was a popular destination for the "knife and gun club" on Chicago's west side. Our service oversaw the vascular service as well, meaning that the surgical cases were especially intense, especially if a knife or bullet severed an artery.

THE DOG LAB

Surgery Grand Rounds took place once a week, and it proved to be a time of extreme stress for the residents. They were in a pyramid, and everyone was afraid they wouldn't be back the next year. This raised the bar on the quality of the presentations, because the residents were literally competing with each other.

I watched my own resident, we'll call him Red, get torn to shreds by the attendings after he presented a case that he had operated on a few days earlier. It was brutal and not a pretty sight to behold. It seemed that they did that to whoever was presenting. Big stick, little carrot.

When grand rounds ended, I ran into one of the other students as I was walking out the door.

He said, "Jesus. Hope he doesn't kill himself tonight. He's your resident, right?"

I responded protectively, "Yes he is. Red is actually a pretty good guy. I feel really bad for him."

"Maybe he should've spent more time in the Dog Lab."

I looked at him, horrified. "What the hell is the Dog Lab?"

"You don't know about that? I thought everybody did."

"No, maybe we don't all know about it. What is it?"

He looked at me smugly, saying, "Well, it's over at County. It seems that they get a lot of large dogs from the pound that were going to be euthanized. Instead, they bring them over to the surgical department so we can practice."

"What do you do to these dogs?"

"Well, we anesthetize them, of course, and then we practice different types of surgical procedures, you know like bowel resections, vascular repairs, and all that stuff."

"Then what happens?"

"While they are still asleep, we inject a lot of air into their veins until they just die."

I didn't know what to say to him, I just kept walking. Maybe I'm weak, but I really could never bring myself to do that to a dog. Some of my best friends have been dogs.

Lesson Learned: Adopt pets from pounds.

THE YELLOW LADY

Early in my surgical rotation, a woman was admitted through the ER with obstructive jaundice. She was bright yellow and her belly was distended with fluids due to liver failure. By now, I was no stranger to liver failure.

To understand this condition, you need to know that the liver produces bile, which passes down the left and right hepatic ducts. Once the bile is south of the gall bladder, it travels through the common bile duct into the bowel. Any obstruction to the flow of bile can produce a backup. Since the liver removes the byproducts of dead blood cells, any backup will cause more of the yellow pigment to accumulate. If you have a significant blockage of this system, you will turn yellow; the technical term is jaundice.

I followed my intern and resident to the ER as we interrupted our work rounds. It was not an OR day. Even though we were still at a pretty good distance from her, we stopped in amazement. I couldn't believe how jaundiced the patient was... much more than I had seen in our VA liver patients.

Red, the daredevil surgical resident, could only say, "Holy crap!"

My intern, Jack, just stared at her. He turned to me and said, "Have you ever seen anything like this before?"

I thought for a moment, trying to sound intelligent, and said "No. This is more dramatic than the cirrhosis I've seen at the VA."

Red turned to Jack and said, "This has gotta be an obstructed bile duct. It's gotta be a stone or cancer."

We walked over to the lady's bed. Red introduced himself and the rest of us.

He asked her, "Is it okay if we examine you?"

She looked at him and then the rest of us with her bright yellow eyes, with a confused expression. It took her a few minutes to process the question and then she nodded.

Red pulled back the cover to expose her abdomen and we all took a breath. There was a long, fresh incision going across her entire abdomen. In those days, gallbladder surgery required a large incision and it looked something like this one, but not exactly.

Because of her bulging belly, some of the stitches had broken and there was a combination of clear fluid and pus coming from parts of the wound. Red motioned for us to follow him away from the bed.

He was incredulous. "Holy shit!" "Who the hell butchered her?"

Jack had the chart in his hand. "She's never been admitted here..."

"Damned right! Listen," he said, aimed especially for my benefit, "This looks like a botched gallbladder surgery. She probably has complete obstruction of the common duct and, obviously, she has liver failure. Look at the ascites..."

Ascites is fluid that accumulates in the abdomen, caused by severe liver damage. Sometimes a person with liver disease will accumulate a few liters of fluid in their abdominal space.

Red looked at both of us, saying, "We're going to be here all night. Let's admit her and get things moving. Chop chop."

The phrase "chop-chop," coming from a surgeon, was amusing. He actually said it, as I clearly recall.

We called all the hospitals in the area and no one had heard of her. We had no idea where her surgery was performed.

I went into her room to see if she could tell me anything. She was very confused because of the condition known as hepatic encephalopathy. In severe liver failure, the impuritics in the blood, including ammonia, can cause swelling of cells in the brain. In time, this leads to hepatic coma.

The poor woman didn't even know where she was and she was unable to tell us an address or even her last name. As a result, we were unable to notify any family members.

I recall seeing her on rounds when we got her to the floor, bleeding from her gums and oozing blood from the slightest bruise. She was struggling to breathe because the fluid accumulating in her belly had pushed up her diaphragm. She could only take short breaths.

She went downhill fast; nothing worked to save her. We drained some of the ascites fluid from her belly so she could breathe easier, but she died that night.

The autopsy showed that her common bile duct had been stitched closed! Red told us he had heard rumors of a quack surgeon somewhere in the Chicago area who was doing weight loss surgery in his basement. Perhaps he was doing a primitive form of bypass surgery and accidentally tied off the common bile duct. Our attendings were furious and notified the police. I never heard whether they found the person responsible.

Lesson learned: Never trust a doctor who performs surgical procedures in a basement.

DIDN'T I SHOOT YOU?

One of my surgical residents was a Chinese-American from San Francisco. I'll call him Dennis. He was a good surgeon, and he was very aggressive when it came to treating surgical problems. I learned a lot from him, and I learned not to sit on things that I might regret later.

One day we had to go over to the VA to evaluate an older man with possible gallbladder disease. The patient was an old WWII veteran who was a chronic alcoholic with significant dementia. He reminded me of the typical patients I was seeing while on physical diagnosis at the VA.

Dennis and I walked into the room and started to ask a few questions. The patient had slurred speech and didn't make a lot of sense, so we went directly to the physical examination. As Dennis was palpating the man's abdomen, the man looked up and said, "Didn't I shoot you in the Philippines back in '44?"

I looked over at Dennis, expecting him to be insulted. He was laughing.

"No, I'm pretty sure you didn't. Besides, I'm not Japanese."

Dennis was a hell of a good sport, and he indeed took out that man's gallbladder. A few weeks later, the man was discharged, probably so he could continue to drink himself to death. He must've seen a lot of hell in the Philippines.

Lesson learned: Don't feel insulted when a demented person picks on you.

THE STABBING AND THE KITCHEN KNIFE

Night call was interesting on general surgery. We were responsible for our service, as well as for the service that went home to try and sleep. If anyone spiked a fever or had any post-op problems, we were on it. If the ER called, we were on it.

Food was never a problem. Usually one of the nurses or orderlies or a lowly medical student would go on a food run. A common staple on the on-call diet was the Fontano's sub. You may recall, I was introduced to these culinary masterpieces by the Cook County ER staff. To this day, including my growing up in New

York and New Jersey and living in Europe, these are by far the finest sandwiches I have ever eaten.

One of the orderlies made the trip to West Polk Street and brought back an armload of those long sandwiches, like a person would carry a load of logs for a fireplace. Once they were distributed and the proper change given back to each person, the med students and residents would retreat to the chart room. We would try to eat in peace unless a crisis arose... and they commonly did. You could always rewrap the sub and stash it for later. You can't do that as well with a pizza.

It was a Friday night, and the wild people of Chicago were getting wilder. When a stabbing victim arrived in the ER, we were off on a new quest.

Surgeons like to operate, so when there is any occasion where there is a potential surgery, they run. It has nothing to do with money; it has to do with getting cases for their credentialing. Just as struggling actors accumulate a reel of their noteworthy performances, so does a surgical resident need to get more notches on their case list.

Red, Jack, and I ran down the steps to the ER. The patient was a young black male with a one-inch wide stab wound in the left upper quadrant of his belly. When we took away the pressure dressing, there was a pulsating ooze of blood.

Red looked the man in the face, and in his direct way said, "I think they must've gotten an artery."

We checked his blood pressure lying and sitting up to see if pressure dropped or pulse accelerated.

Both happened. Jack said, "Major blood volume loss." He turned up the IV to full flow and called the

OR. I started drawing blood for typing and cross matching transfusions, and we hustled to get him into surgery. The other guys were calling the attending and getting the patient to sign a consent form.

For this case, the attending was on his way in, and Jack was asked to scrub in. Being the lowest member on the totem pole, I had to watch the service. In other words, no OR. Bummer.

It seemed like hours before they finally came out of surgery and up to the floor. Red and Jack seemed high as kites. That's what adrenaline does for you. They felt quite proud of themselves.

Red went off to sign some charts, and Jack sat down next to me, grinning.

"So," I asked, "how did it go?"

"Once we got in, I controlled the initial bleeding... the attending let Red and me do the case."

I'm certain that the attending was standing over them like a hawk, because this was such a tricky case.

"The thing about stab wounds is," Jack began reciting, "is that you never know how deep it goes. You have to explore every stab wound."

He was building up some suspense, and I let him enjoy the moment. "So, how deep did it go?"

Red walked over to join in the moment. He added, "Pretty deep, but it missed the splenic artery."

Jack added, "Therefore he must be a dirtball. Only a dirtball would survive a stab wound like that."

He unwrapped the remains of his Fontano's sub and ate ravenously with huge bites. Mine was long gone; I inhaled it while they were in the operating room.

"Yeah," Red agreed, "he's probably a pimp or something."

It was a common belief among the cynical house-staff that dirtballs survive and solid citizens are the ones where stray bullets hit their spine. I must admit that I became just as cynical in the years to come.

Jack continued, "He refused to say who stabbed him, but since it was probably a kitchen knife, there was a good chance it was his old lady. We saw a chick in the waiting room.... She had a pretty nice shiner and it looked fresh. Gotta be an interesting story there."

THE RITUAL OF SURGERY

My initiation into surgery made me think of a sacred ritual, as an anthropologist might describe in a book about primitive tribes.

In the operating room, it looked like a victim was being offered to a high priest, dressed in flowing garb (surgical gown), wearing a sacred hat (surgical cap), wearing a ceremonial mask (surgical mask), and having the victim ritually cleansed and placed before him. He would then take a sacred knife and cut into his victim for the sacrifice...

I'm sure that my surgical friends wouldn't appreciate this analogy, but it was my first impression of a surgical procedure when I finally got to go to the OR.

Because I was the new student on the surgical service, the surgical nurses watched me like a hawk so I wouldn't infect anyone. At that time, the tradition was to go through a detailed and precise scrubbing ritual with a brush and plenty of hot water and soap. Woe be to anyone who might touch the spout of the sink while scrubbing their hands. The nurses would be on you like white on rice and tell you to restart the ritual again.

Once you were properly scrubbed, they would help you put on gloves and a surgical gown. You would have already put on your mask before the scrubbing ritual. Thus cleansed, masked, garbed, and gloved, you walked backwards through the doorway into the operating room, your hands pointing upward from the elbows... Almost like on TV.

As a medical student, you get the distinct impression that you are extremely unwelcome until the nurses get to know you. Most of us sensed a downright hostility if not resentment. We were potential sources of infection that would ruin the case. The student's main job was to stay out of the way. If you were lucky, you might be asked to hold a retractor, although the odds of actually seeing into the operative site were slim.

So it was with surgery, but I really liked it. I loved the drama and the fact that you can actually cure someone. In medicine, including Neurology, we never actually get a cure unless it's a simple infection that responds to antibiotics.

The drama in the operating room is nothing like the idiocy shown on television shows, except perhaps the old TV series M*A*S*H. Contrary to the television scriptwriters, surgeons don't exactly bare their souls to each other in the operating room. Off-color jokes were more the norm in those days before the political correctness fad started.

I didn't get to witness an actual operation until a few days later when someone came in with a hot belly.

MY FIRST SURGICAL CASE

I had just finished drawing some stat bloods when Red came up to me.

"Come on, follow me. We got a hot belly waiting downstairs."

This term was meant to describe a person with severe abdominal pain who might well have a fever and vomiting.

I followed him down to the ER.

"You've been on the service long enough. Go in there and evaluate that patient."

He came in with me but let me do the evaluation.

The patient was a 20-year-old white female, an undergraduate at the U of I Chicago Circle campus. She complained about having a fever and a pain in her right lower abdomen.

Because she had tenderness in the right lower quadrant of her abdomen, an area known as McBurney's point, I pressed down and then released the pressure.

"Ouch!" She yelled.

"I'm sorry. Now I need to gently press on your belly."

Her abdomen was already somewhat tense.

Red motioned me away from the bed. "So, what do you think?"

"I think it might be her appendix." He nodded his approval.

I drew some blood and started an IV, while Red scheduled her for immediate surgery.

He called Jack, who was up on the floor.

"I've got a case for you, Buddy. It's an appy and you can do it. I'll supervise and Messina will be your first assistant."

I overheard what he was saying, and it got me quite excited. The way it usually worked for an appendectomy, the first assistant didn't actually do much more than watch. Red would actually be helping Jack do the case. I didn't care... I was going to the OR!

Remember, in those days there was no particular testing other than clinical examination and a blood count. Today, scanning, ultrasounds, and other techniques would confirm the diagnosis of acute appendicitis, and the procedure would probably be done through a laparoscope, not through a large open incision as we did back then.

As I prepared to go to the operating room, I was scrupulously careful not to anger the scrub nurses. I scrubbed carefully, did not joke or talk, and solemnly followed the resident and the intern into the operating room.

I watched Jack make the incision and describe the anatomy of the structures as he proceeded. My job was to assist with suction or gauze when necessary.

The procedure went well. Red was pleased, and Jack was quite proud of himself. He had already done a good number of this common procedure. As he was preparing to close the skin, he looked up to me and said, "Would you like to close, Doctor?" He already knew about my experience at the Cook County emergency room. Actually, he did all the deep stitches, and he just wanted me to close the skin. A monkey could probably be trained to do it.

I was flabbergasted and nodded up and down. Red apparently had been in on this plan and he said, "Go for it. Use 4-0 silk."

I felt quite secure in my suturing ability, and this was actually quite easy compared to the emergency room. This patient wasn't writhing around, drunk, or screaming. There's a lot to be said for good anesthesia.

Since I first came on the surgical service, I was practicing my knot tying like the other medical students. We practiced like maniacs, using instrument-tying techniques with a needle holder, which we carried in our pockets. We also practiced one-handed knot tying like the surgeons did in the OR. Whenever anyone picked up a telephone on the surgical floor, the telephone wire would have hundreds of small knots made with black suture silk attached to it. We were annoying, but we got better and better at it.

I made my stitches carefully under their watchful eyes. I double-checked each surgical knot, and when I looked up they were both nodding their approval. I felt like a little kid riding my bicycle without training wheels for the first time. It was really no big deal, but it meant a lot to me.

Like I said, I really enjoyed surgery. But then again, I really enjoyed Internal Medicine. I foresaw that I would probably fall in love with every rotation I took. How was I going to make my mind up about my future?

When I finished my basic rotations over the next year or so, I was accepted back as a sub intern on general surgery. Like I said, I liked it a lot and I was thinking very seriously about surgery.

P.L.A.T.O

I had a few days to kill between general surgery and the next clinical rotation, so I spent time in the clinical simulation laboratory. This involves booking time at the P.L.A.T.O. computer.

In the 1970s, computers were not exactly commonplace. The PC was not yet available, and mainframes were enormous. So how was it possible in those days to have a virtual community? We had one.

The University of Illinois medical school prided itself in using innovative technology for training us. The Programmed Logic for Automatic Teaching Operations (P.L.A.T.O.) system is a shining example. It was originally developed by the University of Illinois, Champaign-Urbana, in the 1960s... The 1960s! In those days, the early forms of email, groupware, instant messaging, chat rooms, etcetera, were all part of the P.L.A.T.O system. In truth, I was quite unaware of those features at the time.

The computers were located in the medical school library, and I would go every day in order to sharpen my clinical skills. You see, the P.L.A.T.O. system served as a clinical simulator, which turned out to be of critical importance to me later in life.

It was a primitive looking computer by today's standards, but it actually it had a touch screen. Multimedia was not yet available, but the program allowed me to run recordings to hear heartbeats and turn on devices to see visual images or videos — and it ran in real time.

The program would give me a clinical problem, such as "Mrs. Jones is in your office complaining of abdominal pain. Which of the following steps would you take first?" It would then give me a choice of examining the patient, ordering an x-ray, etcetera. Based on my choices, it would correct me or move to the next step.

Interestingly, the clock was ticking on the corner of the screen. If I spent too long with the problem, it would tell me. At one point, I remember suddenly being interrupted by the program telling me that someone has just collapsed in the waiting room. It asked me what I should do.

This doesn't sound very amazing to those of us who use modern computers, but you must realize this was a true milestone at the time.

THE HEADACHE LECTURE

Although I was able to quiz out of my required medical school courses, I tried to attend lectures that were of particular interest to me.

One such lecture was posted as a special event, presented by the well-known headache expert, Dr. Seymour Diamond. He was the founder of the first private headache clinic and author of hundreds of articles on headache disorders, in addition to many books on the subject. Since I was one of many people in my family with migraine, I decided to attend the lecture, which was held in an amphitheater on the main medical campus.

I was fascinated by what Dr. Diamond was saying about the different types of headaches. Very little was written about this affliction in most of the medical books at that time. I felt that I was in the presence of a true pioneer who was one of a kind. He spoke about migraine and cluster headaches and how people's lives were literally on hold as they suffered from the painful attacks. His research and teaching would affect many thousands of patients over the years, directly and indirectly.

Little did I realize that many years later, I would be a headache specialist in a field that was essentially developed by Dr. Diamond. I am proud to say that he became my friend and colleague and I got to write a chapter in one of his textbooks.

THE WOMEN AND SURGERY

On those days after I completed my general surgery rotation at the University Hospital, while in the midst of intensely using the P.L.A.T.O. system, I would have lunch at the student union each day.

One day I ran into one of my fellow medical students, Connie, sitting in the lunchroom.

"Hey, Connie, how's it going? Mind if I join you?"

She motioned to a chair and I sat down.

"Hey, Ed. What rotation are you on?"

"I just finished general surgery."

She made a face. "How did you like it?"

"Loved it. Have you done surgery yet?"

A disturbed expression crossed her face. "Oh I certainly have."

She went back to eating.

"Connie, didn't you like it?"

It turned out that she was at one of the outlying hospitals that was affiliated with the University of

Illinois. She hadn't been on the service that I was raving about.

She looked up. "It was awful. I suppose the teaching was good, but the surgeons were a bunch of sexist pigs. Assholes."

Hannah had never mentioned this when she was on the University Hospital surgical service, and when I was on my surgical rotation, there were no women, so I didn't see any sexism.

"Why, what do you mean?"

"I mean, all the sexist jokes, the off-color comments ... The surgeons were a bunch of idiots."

"Even the residents?"

"I was on a private service, so it was just me and the attendings."

"You sound disappointed, not just angry."

"I *am* disappointed. Before I started that rotation, I was thinking that I might be interested in being a surgeon. If that was just a taste, I don't think I could handle that for another four years."

She went on to tell me that the changing rooms were in the nurse's locker room section, and the call rooms used by women were located out of the way and far from the floor. In the operating room, she said the surgeons would tell vulgar jokes just to watch her reaction.

They went out of their way to embarrass her. At times, she said, they would brush against her or elbow her in private places when she was stuck holding a retractor during surgical procedures.

The girls in my med school class were tough, but this goes beyond just being tough with adversity. I'm sure these experiences affected the girls in my class, but maybe it wasn't as bad at the University Hospital.

MICHAEL REESE MEDICAL CENTER

Once I had general medicine and general surgery behind me, I knew that I needed to deepen my knowledge of general Internal Medicine further. At that time, I still didn't know what my specialty would be, but I knew that I wanted to spend a lot of time at Michael Reese Hospital.

As I said earlier in this book, Michael Reese had been a premier teaching hospital. It was a famous place where the electrocardiograph was perfected, the gastroscope was developed, and important diabetic discoveries took place. The hospital was the first to have an infant incubator for their newborns and premature babies.

I knew the area well. I went to graduate school at the Illinois Institute of Technology, which was right down the street from Michael Reese. The neighborhood had been declining since World War II, and Michael Reese Hospital as well as the Illinois Institute of Technology decided not to abandon the area. Their plan was to try to acquire property and gentrify the area. In later years, they learned that it was not going to work.

Michael Reese had an extensive campus. At its height, the hospital had 2,400 beds and was the largest hospital in Chicago. They had about 1,000 beds when I was there, considerably larger than the University of Illinois Hospital.

In addition to the main buildings for ward medicine, private medicine, surgery, pediatrics, etcetera, other buildings housed a tumor center, the Psychosomatic and Psychiatric Institute, a city public health clinic, a nurse's residence and nursing school, the Segal Institute for Communicative Disorders, the Simon Wechsler Outpatient Psychiatric Facility, and others. It was huge.

I had worked there as a minor administrator, which stimulated me to go to medical school. Now, as a medical student, I wanted to be part of it from the medical side. The teaching at Michael Reese was all done by people with faculty appointments at the University of Chicago. The surrounding neighborhoods had declined to the point where poverty was rampant and the Chicago Projects were not far away. It was a perfect environment for learning medicine.

Thanks to my flexibility with the James Scholar program, I signed up for a rotation outside of the usual University of Illinois system. During this eight-week Internal Medicine rotation, I would be the only University of Illinois student; the others came from the University of Chicago medical school.

With my experience from the first medicine rotation, I dove into my Internal Medicine reading energetically. I would essentially be competing with students from the prestigious University of Chicago.

In those days, the standing joke was, "How can you tell a University of Illinois student from a University of Chicago student?"

The answer was, "The University of Chicago student can quote the latest medical literature about their patient but the University of Illinois student can tell you their blood count, latest blood chemistries, and their cardiogram."

I felt confident that I had a practical approach to medicine and I felt good that I could read intensely before the new rotation started. This was going to be more academic, and I felt it would round me out.

I was assigned to the Meyer House Pavilion. This was a private building for private patients, and on some floors they even had their own chef who had previously appeared on the cover of Time magazine. The building was situated so the patients could look out their windows and see beautiful Lake Michigan.

The pace for a medical student on the private service was a little slower than the charity wards in the Main Reese building, but the teaching was more intense because of the severity of the patients.

My intern was Mary. She was smart, but not condescending, and she enjoyed teaching. I felt welcomed from the start, maybe because she had also gone to the University of Illinois medical school.

It was quite a cultural shock for me to have gone from minor administrator to medical student. When in the cafeteria, I would run across old colleagues who ran the different hospital departments. It was quite convenient, I must say, when I needed special help from medical records or the laboratory. It always amazed my residents that I could get charts or lab test results so quickly.

FOOTBALL HELMETS AND BLEEDING

Perhaps because I had a previous medicine rotation, Mary asked me to help her with several cases that needed more attention than the others did. One of them was a man with esophageal varices. Esophageal varices develop when liver disease blocks blood flow to smaller vessels, causing protruding veins in the lower part of the esophagus. These are most commonly found in drinkers who have liver disease. These varices are quite dangerous because they can produce significant upper G.I. bleeding.

I told Mary that I had no experience with esophageal varices, so she showed me a few tricks. Endoscopy was not yet perfected for this problem, so more primitive methods were necessary. She smiled as she led me into the room where the man was, waiting for my reaction. He was a middle-aged white executive who seemed quite heavily sedated. He was wearing a football helmet.

Mary laughed when she saw my expression and then explained that he was an alcoholic and they were sedating him with a drug called Librium so he wouldn't go into the DTs.

"Okay," I asked "but why the football helmet?"

She chuckled. "The patient has bleeding esophageal varices, so we put a tube down his nose into his stomach which has a balloon at the end. The idea is to pull up on the tube just enough so the balloon will compress the bleeding veins around the entrance of the esophagus.

"Because he is somewhat confused, like many of these patients, we use the helmet to attach the tube at the right tension."

He indeed had a red rubber tube coming out of his nostril, which passed through the face guard of the football helmet and attached to a bag of water hanging at the side of the bed.

Mary pointed to the bag.

"This provides the traction, and he can't pull it out so easily."

They say that necessity is the mother of invention, and it was certainly true in this case.

"Now," she said, "here's the bad part. I want you to stay at bedside for a while and do some ice water lavage."

"What's that?" I was already not liking this.

"Here, I'll show you."

She took a large Toomey syringe and stuck it into a bucket of iced salt water, sucking up the freezing cold liquid. She attached it to the tube that ran down the middle of the balloon tube and squirted it down.

"You give it a few seconds and then you suck it back up again."

She demonstrated this, bringing up a reddish liquid, no doubt from his bleeding. She then squirted it into a receptacle.

"Here, you try."

It wasn't exactly rocket science.

"This man has ulcers as well as esophageal varices and the idea is for the cool water to constrict the blood vessels. There's also a theory that it slows down the enzymatic breakdown of the stomach wall. Why do you think it's important to pull out the blood?"

I thought for a moment. "So that it doesn't become digested?"

"Bingo. This guy already has high ammonia levels from his bleeding, making him pretty confused.

I'm sure that at the present time, Mary has much better ways of treating G.I. bleeding. I don't believe that this has been part of the treatment plan in recent years, but it seemed to work back then.

THE MAN WHO DIDN'T HAVE A LEFT SIDE

One morning during work rounds, we learned that a new patient was being directly admitted to our service. The man was a private patient of a well-known private internist, Dr. Edward Newman, so he was admitted directly to the medicine floor. He arrived just before rounds so no one had examined him yet. Dr. Newman had arranged for the admission based on the patient's wife calling with her concerns. That was all we knew.

Paul, my intern, pulled me aside. I could see his frustration with the appearance of a totally new patient. He was already overloaded and was trying desperately to catch up. Since it was a private service, he had to deal with many demanding well-to-do patients. It was a stark contrast to the charity floor on the other side of campus. Poor people didn't try to second guess us.

He said, "Ed, here is your big chance to see someone totally new to the service. I want you to really find out what's going on with this guy. If you have any problems, come and get me."

At first, I felt flattered, but then I realized that he was essentially dumping on me. After I had laboriously gathered a detailed history to create my own note, he would then go over it, take out the high points, confirm them, and write his own note. I didn't care. This is going to be interesting.

Mr. Kaplan, we will call him for the sake of privacy, was an overweight white executive in his mid-50s who was lying quietly in bed facing his wife who was sitting on his right. She looked worried and she was holding his right hand. They both looked up when I walked into the room. I smiled and walked around to the opposite side of the bed so I could face both of them.

"Hello," I began, "my name is Ed Messina and I'm a medical student on this service. They've asked me to talk with you and gather information for the rest of the team."

Mr. Kaplan didn't look at me. He kept looking at his wife.

"Isn't the doctor coming in?" She asked me, somewhat disappointed.

"I'll be the first of several people to examine your husband. Dr. Newman is on his way in."

I pulled up a chair on the opposite side of the bed from her.

"But first, I need to ask a few questions."

Mr. Kaplan ignored me. He didn't appear interested in talking to me or answering any of my questions. His wife looked worried and took over.

"I'll try to help as much as I can," she said.

By now, I was used to the fact that a medical student isn't usually taken seriously, so I took in stride the fact that Mr. Kaplan was ignoring me.

Mrs. Kaplan, on the other hand, was quite pleasant and attentive, and seemed to understand the process. Her husband looked at her and smiled. He didn't seem at all troubled that his left arm wasn't moving. It was as if he couldn't hear me.

"Okay. Thank you. When did this all begin?"

"It happened last night," she said, reaching over and picking up his limp left arm. "I think he was trying to get out of bed because he fell and woke me up. It was then that I noticed his left arm wasn't working because he couldn't get up from the floor without my help."

"What did you do?"

"I called Dr. Newman, our internist. He told me to call an ambulance and come directly to the hospital."

Mr. Kaplan had been seeing Dr. Newman for high blood pressure and diet controlled diabetes. His wife said that these had been under good control. She was worried that he had had a stroke since his left arm didn't move and his left leg was weak as well. He was unable to walk by himself.

We spoke at length, and I took notes about his entire past medical history and any symptoms he might've had, according to his wife. She would re-ask him questions that he ignored coming from me, and then he answered them. It appeared that he still did not wish to talk to me, and this seemed somewhat puzzling to Mrs. Kaplan. I guess he usually wasn't so rude.

"He doesn't seem to think there's anything wrong," she said, worried. "Do you think this is psychological?"

"I'm sorry; I think it's too soon to know. Let me do my examination first."

"Okay. While you do that, I'll go out to the lobby and have a cigarette."

She kissed him on the cheek and he responded, smiling.

He spoke, saying, "Come back soon, honey."

I came around the bed to the right side of the bed, the classic place to do an examination, and he looked up at me, surprised.

"Well hello, I didn't know the doctor was in the room."

Puzzled, I explained to him who I was and what I wanted him to do. He was most pleasant and cooperative.

I looked into his eyes with my ophthalmoscope and asked him to follow my finger to the right, and I didn't notice any problem. Asking him to follow my finger in the opposite direction, I noticed he was unable to follow my finger to the left of midline. I also noticed that there was a slight droop to the left side of his face. When I wiggled my fingers in his right visual field, he acknowledged them, but he did not acknowledge any movement from his left field of vision.

When I asked him to lift both arms in front of him, his right arm came up without difficulty. His left arm stayed at his side. I reached for it and found that it was heavy and limp. It seemed not to bother him.

"Mr. Kaplan, can you raise your left arm?"

"I am. Can't you tell?"

I became even more puzzled. I continued my examination and had the same experience with his left leg. I didn't dare get him up to walk. I walked around to the other side of the bed and asked him some questions. He ignored me again. This was indeed a mystery.

I came around to the right side of the bed and completed the rest of my neurological examination, and then I examined his heart, lungs, and the rest of the general exam.

When I came out of the room, Paul the intern rushed in. "You done?"

"Yeah, what's going on?"

He looked stressed. "Dr. Newman called for a private neuro consult from the Chairman of Neurology.... You know, Dr. Klawans, and he's on his way now. You'd better write up this case because YOU are going to present the patient to him." He disappeared into the room.

This was an unusual situation. Certainly in a teaching hospital such as Michael Reese, every admission is worked up by the medical student, the intern, the resident, and then the attending. Every patient...private or not. I later learned that Mr. Kaplan's company gave generous gifts to the hospital. Michael Reese, in those days, was very well funded.

I rushed over to the nursing station and began writing my note as quickly as I could. The resident came over and gave me a malicious smile.

I sensed that it was his perverse sense of humor when he said, "I want to be sure you understand. *YOU* are presenting your findings on a big shot to the most demanding Neurology attending in the city. He's gonna eat you for breakfast and spit out your bones like an owl. I'm glad this is not me." He walked away chuckling.

As I scribbled, I wondered if he was kidding. I knew Dr. Harold Klawans's reputation from my days working at Reese before medical school, and he was truly a national figure. He was only ten years older than I was, and he already had 200 publications to his credit. Although I had only met him at administrative meetings, he seemed to be quite outspoken with his powerful voice. That voice...

With only minutes to spare, I frantically found the copy of *Harrison's* which I kept in my briefcase. I hurriedly tried to find the stroke section. I still didn't have a good enough handle on what was wrong with Mr. Kaplan.

As I almost found something helpful, Paul rushed into the room.

"Come on! Let's get to the conference room. Stat."

I hurriedly put my white coat back on, straightened my tie, and rushed to the conference room.

Around the long table sat my three fellow medical students, my intern, and resident. The illustrious and snappily dressed Dr. Newman-the-society-doctor was grinning... and there was Dr. Klawans.

He was smiling and nodded pleasantly to me, acknowledging that he recognized me from my previous life at the hospital.

His demeanor then changed and he said, in booming tones, "So who's presenting this patient?"

I raised my hand and I felt the eyes of the other students on me. It was quite competitive between students in that service; everyone would try to hot dog each other by throwing out bits of knowledge during rounds, which would give hints at how much they had been reading. It was called roundsmanship.

I was in no mood for that nonsense today. I just wanted not to become a breakfast tidbit. I ignored the other students and began my droning litany in true case presentation style.

" ... The patient is a 55-year-old, right-handed white male with diabetes and hypertension. He was admitted because of his wife's observation that he was unable to move his left arm and leg."

I paused for effect (or maybe it was fear for what I was about to say).

"Mr. Kaplan is unaware of his deficit and he seemed to ignore me when I was on his left side."

I could hear one of the bowtie-wearing U of C students chuckle. He was a bit full of himself, as I had previously observed. I looked up to see what Dr. Klawans would say.

"Excuse me," the booming voice said. "Would you repeat that, please?"

Oh, shit, I said to myself. Here it comes... in the great medical tradition of teaching through intimidation.

"I said that Mr. Kaplan is unaware of his left-sided deficit."

Dr. Klawans jumped to his feet. "Come on, let's go to bedside."

I led the way as the group filed out of the room and down the hall. Dr. Klawans stopped us at the door and peeked inside, waving to Mr. Kaplan. He quietly closed the door and turned to us.

"I want you all to get on the left side of the bed," he said. Then, pointing at me, "Ed, you and I will stand on his right side."

When we were in position, he had me describe my physical findings and nodded politely as I spoke. While I was talking, he was listening to me but also was concurrently doing his own neurological exam. Dr. Klawans wasn't malignant at all. He was actually quite Socratic as he drew out, through his questions, my explanation of the neurological findings. He walked me through my explanation of the anatomy and vascular supply of the frontal and parietal lobes of the brain.

He was grinning at this marvelous teaching activity. He was a superb showman and it appeared not to be at my own expense. He loved a good teaching case. My goal in life is never to *become* a good teaching case... or any kind of interesting patient, for that matter.

He handed the patient a piece of paper and said, "Sir, would you kindly draw me a clock with the numbers that show the hours?"

He held the paper down onto the patient's tray table so it would not slide, knowing that the patient's left arm was not going to be much help. The patient gave him a puzzled look but complied. When he was done, Dr. Klawans took the paper and held it up for everyone to see.

Instead of a round circle with evenly spaced numbers from one to 12, Mr. Kaplan drew the right half of a clock. It looked like an uppercase "D." He crowded all the numbers in the right side of the half circle, so that the twelve was where the six would normally be.

Dr. Klawans leaned over the bed and said, "Mr. Kaplan, you have what we call spatial neglect... the left side of space does not exist for you. It's from a stroke. Please excuse me while I confer with the other doctors, I'll be back soon and we'll talk about this some more."

He excused himself and motioned for the entourage to leave the room. The group that was on the patient's neglected side caught Mr. Kaplan's attention as they passed into his good visual field and filed out of the room. He wasn't aware that they had been there.

In the hallway, Dr. Klawans gave a mini-lecture on this rare but fascinating stroke syndrome. He told me that my localization of the lesion was correct. I felt quite good about the whole encounter, but felt bad for poor Mr. Kaplan.

In later years, I worked extensively with Dr. Klawans in the clinic, and he even sponsored one of my research projects from his departmental budget when he moved to Rush. He wrote an influential letter of recommendation, which helped get me into the residency of my choice. He was a marvelous clinician and teacher, and I mourned his passing in 1998. He was influential in my choice of Neurology as a specialty.

THE GIRL WHO WAS TOO SMART

When I was a student on the Medicine service, one intern did not have any students assigned to her for reasons I learned later. Let's call her Suzie.

Suzie was brilliant. She had several of her completed research studies published when she was still a medical student at a prestigious university. The problem was that she was unable to organize her work. She was not as practical or efficient as an intern needed to be. For example, on a typical call night, a Medicine intern could admit at least six patients from dinnertime until the following breakfast, often as many as 12. I use mealtimes as a unit of measure since time otherwise had no meaning to us.

When we came in to make rounds in the mornings, Suzie would be just finishing her second admission for the night; at least four more had not been seen yet. Of course, to the dismay of the other interns and medical students, we would have to pick up her slack in addition to our own work. The patients needed to be worked up no matter what.

Suzie never saw daylight. She slept sparingly in the Nurses Dormitory where she lived. She would travel to her room through the complex Michael Reese tunnel system, never going outside. She was always working and never playing; not that there was a lot of spare time anyway.

One day when she was on the ER rotation and a patient was brought in with a full cardiac arrest, she had to manage the code... the rest of the staff were busy with another arrest.

According to the scuttlebutt, she pushed the wrong medicine into the IV and the patient died. People said that she subsequently fell into a deep crying depression and had to be admitted to the Psychiatry service. She never returned to complete her internship. People said that she ended up in research, where she was probably better suited.

The Michael Reese medicine internship was tough on people. Still, as crazy as it may sound, I wanted desperately to become a Michael Reese medical intern.

THE MICHAEL REESE NEUROLOGY STUDENT ROTATION

I was so impressed with Dr. Klawans that I signed up for a short, one-month Neurology rotation in the month before my OB Gyne rotation started. Little did I know that I'd be back for more.

The Neurology residency-training program at Reese was in its infancy, so I followed Dr. Klawans on teaching rounds. We had a full neurological service on the first floor of the Meyer House pavilion where interesting people were admitted, charity or not.

When things got busy, I would do admissions and work on the inpatient floor as well.

MOVIE STARS

Late one afternoon, I was covering the inpatient Neurology floor with the Neurology resident. There were several admissions. As I was helping the resident draw blood on the last admission, the ER called our floor. I could see that my resident was exhausted, and when he hung up, he looked like he was going to cry. We would get that way sometimes, when there was no hope of ever getting a decent night's sleep or a hot meal.

He said tiredly, "Ed, go down to the ER, they've got a John Doe down there with a stroke."

With my best "confident" voice I said, "No problem. I'll take care of it." The poor resident definitely needed a break.

In medicine, when an unidentified person is brought into the hospital they are known as either John Doe or Jane Doe.

When I got down to the ER, I saw an elderly black man lying on the gurney. He looked to be in his 70s, but he couldn't speak or move his right arm. He had no ID on him, and he couldn't tell me who he was.

I completed a full examination and initiated orders that later would be cosigned by my poor resident. The man was sent up to the floor after making his circuitous trip through the tunnels.

I got to the floor before the patient did. I presented the information about John Doe to my resident.

"It was pretty straightforward. Right hemiplegia and aphasia."

He nodded.

When a stroke occurs on the left side of the brain, there is paralysis on the right side of the body. Most right-handed people — and some left-handed people — have their speech center on the left hemisphere of the brain. For this reason, a large stroke in the left hemisphere will take away the person's speech as well as their ability to move their right arm and leg.

John Doe understood that I was trying to help him. He smiled at me warmly, although I knew he was scared to death. To this day, it breaks my heart when I see someone with this type of stroke.

The next morning when I dragged myself onto the floor, half asleep, I noticed that the nurses were all talking among themselves and some of them were giggling. Everyone was standing in the hallway. Several security guards were standing around the floor as well; sarcastically, we used to refer to them as "Michael Reese's Finest." There was something in the air and I was curious.

I walked into the nursing station and started loading my charts onto the little pushcart we would use to carry the charts from room to room on rounds. When I picked up the chart for John Doe, I stopped in my tracks.

There was a huge, front-page newspaper article taped to the front of John Doe's chart. It turned out that he was a famous movie star. Someone must've tracked him down and called the emergency room last night. Although this all appeared in the newspaper and there is mention of this on the IMDB.com (The Internet Movie Database) we will respect John Doe's privacy in this book. For this reason, I will keep referring to him as John Doe.

What was interesting to me was the fact that he was so beloved by the people in Hollywood. He was one of the first black movie stars, but in recent years he had fallen onto hard times. Based on what the newspaper said, he seemed to have dropped out of the limelight years earlier.

Word of his illness reached Hollywood rapidly — literally overnight.

My resident had not come to the floor yet, and the nurses said that he was doing a consult with Dr. Klawans elsewhere in the building. He left a message telling me to start rounds without him. Despite the previous night's multiple admissions, the service was actually pretty small.

I was fine with that, and as I started pushing my little cart from room to room, the head of security came up to me.

"Doc, you know we have a celebrity here on the floor?"

"Yes, I know. Why all the guards?"

"We need to keep the press out of here. Also," he looked around furtively, "there are some big shot celebrities coming to visit him today."

"So, how does that affect us?"

"Well, here's the deal. We heard that John Wayne is coming this morning, probably on his way right now. We heard that he flew in last night."

"Well, that's pretty cool."

"Yeah, but the press is going to mob him. I'd like to ask a favor of you."

"Shoot." I was getting a little impatient because my resident was going to give me a hard time if I didn't finish rounds soon.

"I just want you to keep him off the floor so nobody bothers him. The president of the hospital wants to come by and meet him later."

"Now there's a treat for any celebrity." I said, sarcastically. I don't think he got my sarcasm.

Michael Reese Hospital was no stranger to celebrities, and the security department was quite experienced with how tenacious the press was.

I assured the security guard that I would do my best, and I pushed on to make my rounds. Ironically, the next patient on my rounds was John Doe. When I listened to his chest, it didn't sound that great, so I ordered an urgent chest x-ray. I was concerned that he might have choked on his own secretions and maybe was developing pneumonia.

On rare occasions, the gears and the cogs of the universe mesh perfectly. In less than a half-hour, an orderly was wheeling John Doe down to x-ray. I took the precaution of ripping the newspaper article off the front of his chart before they took it. He was still listed as John Doe. The man deserved peace.

I must admit that I really wanted to meet The Duke. I had seen most of his many movies. He was a national hero, and indeed a true film icon.

I was moving along quickly on my rounds when the nurses called me to the telephone. It was my resident.

"Hey Ed, I'm still stuck in the ER waiting for somebody to come in. There is some kind of political bullshit, so I need to stick around down here. How are you doing up there?"

"Things are under control here."

I selfishly didn't tell him about John Wayne. I wanted to be the one to meet him.

"Well, I appreciate your help up there. You're okay. I'll catch you later."

I didn't feel guilty.

The charge nurse came up to me, saying, "Listen, John Doe is going to be in x-ray longer than we thought. Apparently, there were some emergencies, so x-ray is tied up for the moment. I just hung a fresh IV before he left, so it won't go dry. It would be nice to give him something by mouth, don't you think?"

I was beginning to learn that nursing suggestions should never be ignored. It makes your life much easier in the end.

"He had a good gag reflex when I examined him, so send someone down to give him some Jell-O." It's hard to choke on Jell-O.

As we were talking, the security detail was ushering John Wayne onto my floor. I could see them down at the end of the hall, and I knew that the towering figure walking between them had to be The Duke.

I walked down to John Doe's empty room just as they reached it. I told the security guys I would take it from here. They looked at each other with puzzled expressions, shrugged, and walked away.

The Duke walked up to me in his characteristic gait, held out his hand and said, "Hiya, Doc."

He looked at the empty bed and then back to me saying "Well, where the heck is he?"

I introduced myself as a medical student, and I asked him to follow me into the small conference room that we used for teaching.

A gaggle of nurses was following us and I asked them to please not let anyone know we were in there.

I looked at their eager faces and said, "Please let me know when he comes back from x-ray."

I closed the door of the conference room and I turned back to John Wayne. He was bigger than life, and I promised myself I would not in any way act star struck or ask him for an autograph.

I offered him some tarry coffee from the coffeepot in the corner, and we sat around the conference table. Since he was able to tolerate that awful stuff, I knew that he really was tough.

"So, what happened to my friend, Doc?" It was nice of him to call me Doc, even though he knew I was just a lowly medical student.

I explained the situation with the stroke and how I was concerned about pneumonia.

"You know, Doc, that man has helped a lot of us in the old days. When we were struggling young actors, he was like a superstar, but he was a good guy. For those of us who worked in pictures in the '30s, that racial crap was no big deal. I know he caught a lot of static from a lot of people because of the parts that he played."

John Wayne's conversational speech style was identical to the way he spoke in movies. For a moment, I felt like I was on the set of *Sands of Iwo Jima* or *Rio Bravo*.

He explained to me that he had a slight acquaintance with the medical world since his dad had been a pharmacist.

"Also, you know, I had lung cancer a few years ago. I think I might've just beaten it."

This is the man who was quoted for saying, "I licked the Big C."

As we spoke, I told him that John Doe was on a ward service, which is a charity service.

"Well, that's got to stop. You know in Hollywood we take care of our own. I heard Ben Vereen is coming out later today. We'll figure a way to fly our buddy back to Hollywood. He's one of us, and we'll treat him that way."

We must've been talking for about 20 or 30 minutes before the charge nurse knocked on the door. She opened the door and stuck her head in, smiling broadly at our celebrity guest.

"He's back in his room now."

Within hours, John Doe was on a private flight back to Hollywood where his friends were going to take care of him. Later that year he won the NAACP Special Image Award for his pioneering movie career.

My resident, who was somewhat of a film buff, was furious when he found out what he had missed. *C'est la vie, mon ami.*

THE SURGEON WHO COULDN'T CUT STRAIGHT

While I was on the Michael Reese Neurology service, there was a new admission that seemed to make everyone uncomfortable. I heard about it secondhand from one of the other students who was on call for the first floor, Meyer House Pavilion. I was on the consult service with Dr. Klawans so I followed him into the patient's room.

The patient was a well-known general surgeon; we'll call him Dr. Schwartz. He was admitted for evaluation of a neurological problem, and he was scared to death. When some surgeons are frightened, they act mean as a defense.

The previous day while beginning a routine laparotomy in the operating room, he started to make his first incision, and his scalpel made a zigzag. He was so disturbed by this that he let his assistant take over and he supervised.

The surgeon looked at both Dr. Klawans and I as we walked into his room. He of course knew Dr. Klawans, but he looked at me suspiciously. I introduced myself as a medical student. At first, I thought he would ask me to leave, but he smiled and simply said hello to me with kindly smile. I could tell he was trying hard. We were at a teaching hospital, and he graciously accepted that fact.

Dr. Klawans took a careful history. He asked his questions so skillfully that I don't think the patient even suspected that he was being interrogated. Apparently, they were old friends from medical school. Dr. Schwartz said that he had been noticing some clumsiness recently, but never to the point where it affected his patients, he hastened to add. On the day in question, when he tried to make the incision, he was shocked to find that he couldn't control his hand. Dr. Klawans continued taking the history, the patient noting that several years earlier, he had double vision for a few days but he was on vacation and didn't tell anyone. It got better in about a week. I think deep inside, he knew something was going on, but denial is a powerful force in medicine, and we doctors are the worst patients.

We did a careful neurologic examination and found that Dr. Schwartz had difficulty bringing his finger to touch his nose and then out to the examiner's extended finger. Similarly, when we asked him to walk, he had a slight stagger and he was unable to walk like a tight rope walker.

When the exam ended, we stood next to his bed and he looked at both of us. He did not hide his worry.

"You think it's a brain tumor?"

Dr. Klawans told him that there was no way to tell from the examination alone. As I said earlier, the CT scan had not yet become available in Chicago. We sent the patient to the nuclear medicine department for an old-fashioned radionucleide brain scan, and it came back normal.

The old-fashioned brain scan was done by intravenously injecting a radioactive element, technetium. Certain brain tumors would accumulate the element, and a type of Geiger counter would then scan across the person and show areas where there was increased uptake. It was quite imprecise for most uses.

We decided to do a hot bath test. The hot bath test was a somewhat primitive technique in which the patient was brought down to physical therapy and placed in a large sling. A small crane-like device, like a cartoon stork, lifted the sling and swung over to lower the patient slowly into a tank of hot water called a Hubbard tank. A thermometer was placed in the patient's mouth, and when the thermometer read 103 and the patient's face was sweating profusely, the small crane lifted him from the Hubbard tank and onto a nearby stainless steel examination table.

The technique was quite primitive, but the principle was simple. Patients with certain types of white matter disease such as multiple sclerosis will have a different examination when their core temperature is elevated. This is based on the observation that people with multiple sclerosis would often lose neurological function when their body temperature was too high, like on hot days or when they had a fever. They would decompensate.

We examined Dr. Schwartz after he was heated up, and we found that his reflexes became more brisk and his clumsiness became even worse. When we scratched the bottom of his feet, his toes went up instead of down. This is called a positive Babinski test. In summary, he developed additional neurological findings after he was heated up. He also became extremely lethargic during the test; he was unable to talk. When the exam was finished, the surgeon was wheeled back to his room. When he had cooled down and had recovered from the test, Dr. Klawans and I came by to see him.

"Sam," Dr. Klawans said, "I suspect that you might have multiple sclerosis."

Dr. Klawans always said it like it was. He broke the bad news with a smile and in a very supportive way. Dr. Schwartz nodded and looked down at his hands. He looked up at Dr. Klawans, "How sure are you?"

"Well, the best way to prove the diagnosis is to get a spinal tap and look for abnormal immunoglobulin in the spinal fluid.

The surgeon agreed, and one of the residents came by the following morning to do the lumbar puncture. I must say, the resident seemed a bit nervous. Not because he was doing a spinal tap, but because it was on a fellow physician... and on an attending... and on a surgeon.

The fluid was collected and placed into four separate vials, which were sent to the laboratory. These days, we still use spinal fluid analysis but the advent of the MRI scanning has drastically simplified the diagnosis of multiple sclerosis.

Unfortunately, the spinal fluid confirmed the diagnosis of multiple sclerosis. Multiple sclerosis is a condition where the white matter in the brain and in the spinal cord deteriorates because of an autoimmune abnormality. If you think of the white matter in the nervous system as insulation on the wires (nerve cells or axons), then you could imagine how short-circuits could occur between signals traveling amongst the billions of neurons. This can produce paralysis, incoordination, visual loss, and other neurological deficits. Not a good diagnosis for a surgeon. Multiple sclerosis is a degenerative disease, and at the time, no specific medications were available to treat it. Today, we can tremendously slow down the progression of the illness, but we still do not have a cure. At the time of this story, the most aggressive approach was to give intravenous steroids and try to turn off what was assumed to be an abnormal immune response.

I came back the following day and the surgeon had an IV running into his arm that contained a steroid solution. He seemed to be somewhat at peace, although the nurse looked somewhat uncomfortable. I followed her out into the hallway

She looked at me and said, "He's been calling the pharmacy and ordering his own medications. The on-call resident switched them back. I need for you to tell Dr. Klawans."

Indeed, it turned out that the good surgeon was managing his own case, ordering his own IVs and even ordering his own dietary plan. Dr. Klawans was furious, and he went into his room and closed the door to reprimand him. I thought it wise to wait in the hallway. It turned out that the surgeon had a progressive form of multiple sclerosis that was unremitting. During his short stay in the hospital, there was no appreciable improvement or deterioration.

I later learned that, of course, he had to quit surgery at the peak of a very promising career. He didn't handle the news well and adapted very poorly to his role as a patient. Surgeons are very strong-willed individuals and are used to being in charge. When he lost his most precious skill, he lost his interest in medicine and became deeply depressed. I don't know how it finally turned out, but I don't expect it was good.

LIFTING A MAN USING ONLY ONE FINGER

Dr. Klawans was quite famous for his Parkinson's clinic, and he had a huge population of patients who came from a large geographic area. If I recall correctly, the Clinic met each Tuesday afternoon, and it was staffed by all the Neurology attendings and house-staff.

As a homey touch, Dr. Klawans' mother attended and greeted the patients. When people came in to register for their visit, she offered them cookies she had personally baked. It was a very warm and supportive setting; many of the patients had been coming for years and had gotten to know each other.

I went in to see an older man waiting in one of the examination rooms. He was hunched forward on a straight-backed chair with both arms resting on his legs. His hands were hanging down and shaking with what we call a pill rolling tremor. In other words, it looked as though he was rolling a pill between thumb and forefinger on each hand. He had a little bit of saliva drooling down the left side of his mouth, and his face had no expression. It's hard to tell if a Parkinson's patient is sad or whether their facial expression is just a symptom of their illness.

I came closer to him, and a Neurology resident who I will call Dr. Mengal was walking behind and observing me. Before we entered the room, he told me to talk to the man and get him to walk for us.

When I introduced myself, he opened his mouth to speak and his jaw began shaking for a few seconds before a very strained voice was audible. He smiled at me and then slowly reached into his jacket pocket and took out a handkerchief, dabbing at the saliva coming from his open mouth.

As requested, I asked him to stand and show us how he walked.

He nodded in agreement and tried to get up. He leaned forward and was unable to rise, so he slumped back. He tried again and failed, looking helplessly at the two of us.

Dr. Mengal nodded and walked up to him, saying to me, "Watch this carefully."

He pointed his bent index finger to the old man, like a hook.

"Sir, please hook your finger in mine and I'll help you get up."

The old man hooked Mengal's finger with his own, and Mengal effortlessly helped him to a standing position. The man began his slow, shuffling walk across the room, picking up speed. Mengal took his arm and led him back to the chair, thanking him. He turned to me.

"Ed, it's not that he was weak.... He just needed some help with his center of gravity. You could see how he was speeding up as he walked. If he went far enough, he would have gone beyond his center of gravity and fallen forward."

It was in that Parkinson's clinic where I began to deepen my interest in the nervous system. It was a far cry from those impossible brain slices that frightened me on my entrance exam. The brain was where things were happening, and by then I was quite certain that that was the organ I would learn to treat.

THE SEIZURES AND THE SONG

The outpatient general Neurology clinic at Michael Reese catered mainly to the welfare crowd. I was assigned to evaluate a somewhat bedraggled man with a torn jacket. He had epilepsy.

The man told me that earlier that day he had a convulsion while visiting his church, which had services every day. It was one of those storefront churches that you see on the west side of Chicago.

His pastor came with him and said, "It was awful, Doctor. He would just fall to the ground, tense up his body and bite his tongue. Then he started shaking all over; I mean jerking really hard."

I turned to the patient and said, "What was the last thing you noticed before you passed out?"

He thought for a moment and said, "I was standing by the organ, listening to my favorite song."

This pastor interjected, "It was 'Amazing Grace.'"

The man continued. "The next thing I remember was lying on the floor, confused. I didn't know where I was. When I looked up there were all these faces looking down at me. They looked very worried. Gradually I began to recognize who they were. They were my church family."

The pastor stepped in again. "The same thing happens every time he comes to my church. It always happens when he hears them play 'Amazing Grace' on the organ."

I excused myself and went to get my resident to relate this story. The resident smiled and became extremely interested. He asked me to repeat the story in detail and he simply smiled, nodding.

"This is musicogenic epilepsy, I bet." He said.

When I looked at him, puzzled, he continued, "It's a type of reflex epilepsy, very rare, which is triggered by a certain piece of music, usually played on the exact same instrument or by listening to the same exact recording. This is very cool if it's true. Let's go back in there."

He had the man repeat his story, clarifying specific points. Whenever he heard the song, 'Amazing Grace,' the man would have a convulsion. He also had seizures in other settings, but this particular organ playing that song seemed to trigger a convulsion every time. His other seizures didn't follow any type of pattern.

The resident looked at the man, saying, "Sir, I gotta ask you this..."

The man looked at him, waiting to hear what he would say.

"If this song being played on the same organ gives you a convulsion every time, why the heck do you keep coming back?"

I swear to you, the answer the man gave was really as I am telling you. He said, "Because I love that song."

The resident and I looked at each other and then at the pastor. There was no hint of a smile on either of us. I was starting to get good at masking my expressions.

I asked the man, "Are you taking your seizure medicines every day?"

The man looked at his pastor and then back to me. "Well, I do miss a few doses from time to time."

We had a long talk about how important it was not to miss medication doses when you have epilepsy. This pastor told us that he would help the man be more compliant.

We gave him a refill on his prescription and I was about to end the visit and leave the room.

Just then, my smart aleck resident turned toward the man.

"One more thing, sir. If you're out on the street and feel one of your seizures coming on, take your wallet and clamp it in your teeth."

The man nodded and we left the room.

In the hallway, I had to ask my resident the obvious question. "Why would you tell him that? So we wouldn't break his teeth when he clenched down?"

"Oh yeah, that too. No, my main reason was more practical. If he's out on the street in some of these neighborhoods and has a seizure, he'll lose consciousness and probably get robbed. If he clamps the wallet in his teeth, they won't be able to get it from him as easily... Maybe they won't even want to because it'll be full of drool."

OBSTETRICS AND GYNECOLOGY

When I finished my brief taste of the Neurology elective, it was time to begin another one of the required rotations. I chose to do obstetrics and gynecology at Michael Reese because it had a good teaching program and the students had a lot more opportunity to deliver babies. I was thankful for the preparation I received through my brief rotation in the Cook County Hospital gynecology clinic. I felt like I was ready for this new rotation.

The delivery room was the first part of my rotation. Another student and I were assigned to one of the delivery rooms and we observed every delivery, taking turns for days or nights. Like most of the services at Michael Reese, the charity patients and the private patients received equally good care. I was allowed to participate in both types of delivery during my stay.

The plan was for me to observe a number of uncomplicated and complicated deliveries, and it was up to the discretion of the resident or the attending when it would become my turn to deliver some of the less challenging clinic patients.

YOU WORM!

One night, while waiting for the next labor room arrival, I was assigned to one of the private obstetricians, Dr. C, whose practice was on the north side. He tended to cater to the more privileged population, and the only reason they agreed to come down to the south side was because Dr. C was so well known.

A well-to-do yuppie couple was in the labor room, and we were checking the woman at regular intervals. Her contractions were becoming more frequent, and on examination, we knew it wouldn't be long before she would go into more active labor.

Dr. C and I were sitting in the doctor's lounge, waiting. It was a very comfortable room with a couple of nice, comfortable leather armchairs. He was lighting up an expensive cigar and he offered me one. I declined.

"You know, OB is a specialty that requires cigar smoking."

"Why is that?"

"By the time a cigar has burned down, following a certain degree of cervical dilation, the baby will come soon."

I'd like to think that he was kidding, but sure enough, as he stubbed out his cigar after the last puff, the nurses came in and told us the patient was ready for us.

I could hear the usual anguished sounds of a woman in labor, but there was another voice as well. We could hear the husband's anguished sounds of pain as well. Dr. C elbowed me and nodded towards the head of the bed. The poor woman was in the throes of painful labor as we prepared to do a pudental nerve block. Epidural anesthesia was not available. The nerve block allowed at least some pain control while the episiotomy incision was made, to prevent tearing as the baby exited.

The baby was not yet ready to be born at that point, and the woman was experiencing the agonizing pain of labor. Unfortunately, she was tightly gripping the small, pale hand of her husband, and it looked like she was intentionally trying to hurt him. His face was screwed up in pain. He said nothing.

She screamed at him, "You son of a bitch. Look what you've done to me! You've ruined my body!"

He continued to say nothing, but he grimaced with pain as his hand was being crushed in her desperate grip.

The woman's hair was wet with perspiration and her face was drawn back into the expression of combined agony and rage. "I'm never going to be the same! This is all your fault, you worm! You goddamned worm!" She screamed.

This litany of obscenities continued until the labor became more productive and the nurses gave her some anesthetic to inhale through a mask. The delivery continued without incident, and the baby presented normally and appeared normal and healthy. I watched

Dr. C complete the delivery and later stitch up the episiotomy wound.

I was paying close attention to his method of suturing. By the time he was finished, the woman was smiling and pulling her husband down to her pale and sweaty face so she could kiss him. They were both overjoyed with their beautiful little baby girl. I still wonder whether deep inside, the husband somehow resented the pain of his hand being crushed and the lash of the woman's sharp tongue. I speculated that he worked for his father-in-law and had long ago cashed in his testicles.

Lesson learned: Different strokes for different folks.

MAMA MAMA!

The deliveries coming from the clinic population involved women and girls of all ages. The senior OB resident brought me in to observe a delivery.

"After this one, maybe you could deliver the next."

Delivering a baby is one of the most memorable experiences of a medical school career. For reasons as you will see, this patient needed to be delivered by an experienced person, not by a student.

We'll call the patient Renata. This was her second pregnancy. She had miscarried her first baby and she was a personal favorite of my resident, Charlie. Charlie had followed Renata closely during her prenatal visits in the clinic, and he made a point of calling her at home if she failed to show up for an appointment. In the past, Renata had been a heavy drinker and was often unreliable. He told me that she promised him that she wouldn't drink during this pregnancy. She didn't know who the father was and did not care.

Renata was 14 years old, and her mother was with her in the labor room. I don't think her mother was even 30 years old, but she seemed very attentive to her small-framed daughter who looked extremely frightened and was screaming in pain, even in the early stages of labor.

When Renata was ready to give birth, she was wheeled into the delivery room and the pediatrician was asked to stand by. Charlie was concerned that her pelvis was so small that she might need a cesarean section to get this baby out safely. The labor continued, and Renata became more agitated with the pain. The baby seemed to be progressing well through the birth canal, but Renata was frightened and in great pain.

Fortunately, the baby was small enough to pass through her adolescent pelvis, and all was well. What was most memorable about this experience was her constant cries during labor of "Mama Mama, it hurts so bad!"

It was a strange feeling to see the healthy little newborn cradled by this child. Perhaps in another place and time, a Renaissance painter would have done her justice as a black Madonna and child. They were beautiful.

Lesson learned: Age is only relative.

THE NEUROPSYCHIATRIC INSTITUTE

Located next to the old University Hospital, the Neuropsychiatric Institute at the University of Illinois has a long history of research and education. With my developing interest, perhaps obsession, with the brain, I felt that I needed to be well grounded in psychiatry to see if that was where my destiny lay.

The outpatient clinic was laid out in a way that trainees could interview patients individually in small private rooms with one-way mirrors that covered an entire wall. After days of orientation and background training, it was finally my turn to interview a patient.

The interview room had two chairs and a small table with a red telephone on it, known as The Red Phone. I honestly do not recall if it was even red. The instructor sat on the other side of the one-way mirror with the other medical students. He or she would call The Red Phone in the interview room when it was appropriate to change the line of inquiry or to direct and guide the student interviewer.

In those days, psychiatry was well taught because there was an emphasis on interviewing techniques. I still use those skills today. My instructor was an older man; we'll call him Dr. F. He was patient, quiet, and sported a beard that reminded me of Sigmund Freud.

HE WAS ALREADY DEAD!

I'll never forget one of the first patients I interviewed. When I went to get him, I could see him sitting in the waiting room, looking around and scratching his arms repeatedly. He was a very large middle-aged black man from the neighborhood. He looked like he could have been a lineman for the Chicago Bears. He had been sent over by the Dermatology Clinic at County.

He had presented to their clinic with the chief complaint of having bugs or insects jumping out from his skin, and he had badly scratched his skin to the point where it was bleeding. After careful consideration, no doubt with some tongue-in-cheek comments, they found no dermatological or parasitic abnormality. They consequently made a referral to our psychiatry service.

Before I went to get the man from the waiting room, Dr. F said, "With this man, there's probably a strong delusional component, assuming the dermatologists are right and he doesn't have bugs. You might also want to take a look at his arms yourself, just to be sure. If he really is delusional, I want you to ask questions that would help reveal why he has deteriorated from a behavioral perspective. We need to find out what events may have caused him to decompensate."

I nodded and went to the waiting area to lead the man into the exam room. We'll call him Mr. Jones. He followed me into the interview room and took the chair closest to the door. I paused for a moment and then pulled the small table over to the other chair at the other end of the small room. I sat down and pulled The Red Phone next to me. I expected it would probably ring a few times.

I asked him to show me his arms, and he pulled up the sleeves of his sports jacket. There were deep gouges on his large, muscular forearms with scabs in different stages of healing. He scratched them again as we were talking.

I asked him some standard leading questions.

"Why do you think you are here, Mr. Jones?"

He laughed. "The people at County think I'm crazy."

I gave him a classic psych response to that statement, "Do you think you're crazy?"

"Hell no. My problem is insects. Parasites. Look at these arms. Do you mean to tell me that there's nothing wrong?" He was starting to get agitated.

"I understand why you feel that way. Let's just talk a little bit so I can evaluate you and get this thing settled."

"Okay." He sat back, now scratching his belly.

In true psychotherapeutic style, I sat and looked at him, not speaking, to see what he would say next. He looked back at me, scratching his belly. At that point, I was hoping that the dermatologists were correct. I didn't need to catch his bugs or whatever they were. His arms did look somewhat nasty.

We were getting nowhere, just politely looking back and forth at each other, when the Red Phone rang on the table. It startled both of us and I jumped. Trying to appear calm, I picked up the phone and just listened.

Dr. F said, "Ask him if he has ever been in trouble."

This was a good general question. I nodded to the mirrored wall and hung up the phone.

"Sir, have you ever been in trouble... Like, with the law?"

A sly look crossed his face and he smiled. Then he took on a quizzical look and asked me, "You mean, with the cops?"

I nodded.

"Well, there was this one time..."

He proceeded to tell me that he used to have an old Cadillac convertible. One day, he parked it in front of a bar on the West Side, and left the top down when he went inside.

"When I came out of the bar a couple of hours later, there was a man lying across the back seat of my car! I said to myself, what the hell was he doing there? Then, I figured he was probably dead drunk or stoned on somethin'."

I nodded, listening carefully.

"Needless to say, Doc, I was mad and I told him to get the hell out of my car."

"Did he get out?"

"Hell no! He ignored me, so I commenced to beat on him. He wouldn't even wake up. I guess I got carried away... I was hitting him with my gun."

"A gun?"

"Yeah. Then a cop came and arrested me."

"For assault?"

"No, for killing the guy. The cop said he was dead."

I kept a straight face. "So, you went to jail?"

"Only for one night. Turns out, the guy in my backseat was already dead before I was beating on him. The autopsy showed that he died of a drug overdose a couple of hours earlier." He chuckled.

"So, you beat him up with a gun?"

"That's right, Doc. Here it is."

With that, he produced a beautiful Colt Python .357 Magnum revolver from the inside pocket of his jacket.

I could hear scrambling on the other side of the mirror, chairs being pulled back and screeching across the floor. The Red Phone rang. We both startled again, and at that point I realized it wasn't such a good idea to startle the man with the gun. I glared at the mirror.

Fortunately, he wasn't aiming it at me, but the gun was pointing towards the one-way mirror... I imagine that's why I heard the scrambling sounds. They were probably diving for cover. I guess they couldn't tell that his finger was not on the trigger. I didn't perceive it as a threat. He was just proudly showing it to me.

"It's the Rolls-Royce of revolvers." He said, smiling.

I nodded my agreement.

The Red Phone rang again and I picked it up.

My instructor nervously said, "Please tell that gentleman to put the gun away. Do you understand?"

I had to smile as I nodded toward the mirror and hung up the phone. The patient appeared quite harmless and he was not threatening me in any way. I'd certainly been in worse situations than this.

"Mr. Jones, I agree, it's a beautiful piece of work. The problem is, the folks on the other side of that mirror are getting a little bit nervous."

"You mean, the pistol scares them?"

I nodded, "Yeah, my supervisor would appreciate it if you would put your gun away."

"I'm sorry, Doc. I didn't mean to scare anybody. You know that, don't you?"

"I know."

He put away the gun and then turned to wave to the people behind the mirror, followed by a thumbs-up sign. I couldn't control the small chuckle that escaped me.

"So, Doc, what else you want to talk about?"

"What do you do for a living, Mr. Jones?"

"I work as a security guard at a hospital on the south side."

He kept scratching his arms and I also started feeling itchy. We spoke a little bit longer, and honestly,

I couldn't come up with any other delusions. I wondered whether the dermatologist had missed something.

Lesson learned: Not everyone is crazy.

THE SPECIAL FILM

The psychiatry service had many interesting activities. Human sexuality was felt to be in the realm of psychiatry, and the rumor on campus was that a special film was going to be shown in one of the larger conference rooms of the NPI building. What created the buzz was that the film was about a woman inducing her own orgasm. Apparently, someone somewhere had gotten a government grant to produce a clinical film on the topic. I don't believe it was made in Chicago; it might even have been European.

Anyway, the news traveled fast and the small auditorium was packed with students on the day of the showing. I honestly don't know if some of them even brought dates. The film was actually a video with bad sound, and it was obviously made in a laboratory. It was hardly a romantic venue. On the right side of the screen were analog graphics, like an old lie detector test. It showed pulse, respirations, and other parameters as the small pens made their squiggles on the moving piece of paper.

The film itself was not particularly titillating or interesting, but I got a kick out of watching the reactions of the people sitting in the audience. As a rule, the medical students of that era didn't have much playtime, and frankly I don't think a lot of them even dated very much. I got a real kick out of watching my classmates; some were riveted to the screen while others seemed outraged, but they didn't leave.

After the exhibition was over, uncomfortable jokes popped up here and there, and of course, the usual angry indignation from certain people. As I look back on this event, I wonder if the real purpose of the film was to create an attraction as well as a distraction while a hidden camera was filming the audience's reactions. Now, THAT would be an interesting project.

Lesson learned: Watch the watchers.

THE AA MEETINGS

Dr. F was a good teacher and a good psychiatrist. He required all the students on the service to attend courtroom proceedings that dealt with abuse. Space permitting, any citizen can sit in most courtrooms. It was an eye-opener. Spouse abuse takes many forms, and it's often a two-way street.

He also requested that we attend evening Alcoholic Anonymous meetings that were held near the medical campus. AA is a long-standing organization that has helped many alcoholics over many years.

I went each week to the AA meeting with one of my fellow students from the psychiatry rotation. It gave me a much deeper insight into alcohol addiction. We would just go and sit in the back, observing. Sometimes we would munch on the cookies that someone brought in. It seemed like everyone there was puffing on cigarettes. An addiction is an addiction, and many alcoholics who are able to stay on the wagon have tremendous difficulty with quitting smoking. From what I've seen among my patients, I'm convinced that it's harder to quit smoking than it is to quit drinking.

The meetings were informal, and I was struck by how supportive everyone was to the person speaking. The usual opening would be, "My name is_____, and I am an alcoholic." The group, almost in unison would say back, "Hello _____." The person at the podium would then begin telling their story.

People would tell amazing stories, especially those who were there for the first time and who mustered up the courage to finally speak to the group. They often spoke about hitting bottom or the last straw that caused them to quit drinking.

Alcoholism is an illness without a cure, but remissions are possible. To this day, I still send patients to AA when I feel they have a drinking problem. I've never become jaded because I know that some people will find help. I think going to these meetings had something to do with it. You always have to try. That's the lesson I learned from these meetings.

One evening, a man got up. We'll call him Chuck. He stood up in the audience and indicated that he wanted to tell his story. The group clapped, and he stiffly walked up the aisle to the podium. He nervously looked at the group and at first began to stammer. The people in the front row smiled at him and encouraged him to speak.

"Okay, here goes. My name is Chuck and I'm an alcoholic."

"Hello, Chuck," the crowd said.

"I guess I need to tell you how I hit bottom. My story sounds like a lot of the other stories I've heard here. The usual. Too much drinking, eventually getting fired from my job, and then my wife leaving me. Luckily, my house was paid for and my wife was living with her mother until she could decide what she was going to do.

"It was a hot summer's day, and I was trying to mow the lawn. Of course, I already had a good amount of vodka, and the mower was hitting a lot of things. When I rolled it over a rake, the blades stopped and the mower stalled. It ruined the blade. I was crouched on the ground and I tried to flip over the mower to see how bad the damage was. I was swaying a lot and almost fell over."

Chuck looked around the room. The people were listening and there were no other sounds in the room.

He continued. "Well, as I was hunched down on all fours, my cat, Ziggy, jumped onto my back. You know, that's how cats are. You never know what they're gonna do."

The audience laughed. Chuck smiled back.

"Maybe this sounds crazy, but I really started to think about my life. I didn't have any kids and my wife was doing her own thing, but if something happened to me, who would take care of Ziggy?"

The group clapped. He had touched a nerve. The people knew just what he was talking about.

"I mean, it does sound sort of stupid, but that's what it took to make me quit.... At that time. The next thing I knew, I started coming to these meetings."

The group clapped again. Chuck was beaming.

"My last drink was one month ago."

More applause.

"... And I'm gonna make it."

The moderator came up to the podium, clapping, and he shook Chuck's hand, congratulating him. Everyone was smiling. It was a feel-good moment.

As I was walking back to the car after the meeting had ended, I realized that everyone has that one thing that changed his or her life. I was hoping that Chuck could get his life back together again... and keep it that way.

Lesson learned: AA helps people. Never stop sending people.

When the psychiatry rotation was finished, I remained fascinated with the brain, but I was looking for something more physical. I was looking forward to eventually getting my Neurosurgery rotation. So far, Neurology looked very appealing to me, but I needed to see what Neurosurgery had to offer. Before doing any more electives, however, I needed to complete more of my required rotations. The next one was going to be pediatrics.

PEDIATRICS OUT IN THE BURBS

By now, having spent a lot of time in the inner-city hospitals, I thought it might be interesting to do my pediatrics rotation in one of the suburban hospitals. I picked Lutheran General Hospital in Park Ridge, Illinois. Many medical students said that it was a great rotation because the teaching was good and the night call was much less grueling. I admit, I needed a less demanding rotation.

The pediatric experience involved a lot of outpatient exposure in private pediatricians' offices as well as some time in the hospital with the sick kids. No matter where we were, regular conferences were held almost daily that consisted of the students, the residents, and the attending. It was a wonderful rotation because we got to meet all of the subspecialty pediatric attendings such as the geneticist, pediatric surgeons, and others. The conferences were well structured and had very clear objectives.

Once a week, a student would present a case and give a brief talk about the illness represented by the case. During the student conferences, one particular pediatric resident always seemed to have some pearls to share. Let's call him Barry.

By now, having been through some tough rotations, I was feeling salty. Something about Barry was suspicious and I wondered whether he was making up some of the things he was telling the students. Maybe it's because I was older than the other students, but I just had a gut feeling about this guy.

After all, I was used to being around some very high-powered residents in very competitive programs, and this guy was different...there was something about Barry... I got into the habit of looking up things that he was telling us. He would commonly say things like, "...a few weeks ago in the *New England Journal of Medicine*, there was a study about bla bla bla."

When I looked up these tidbits, I was unable to find any corroboration to what he was saying. I had a theory that Barry must've been less than a stellar student, and now as a resident, he could impress the students with his "knowledge." He seemed to keep away from me, perhaps because he could tell I didn't buy his act.

After a couple weeks of this nonsense, a little devil inside of me told me that I needed to do something to embarrass Barry. I'm not a particularly vindictive person, but I had such a high regard for my medical education that I felt it was an affront for people to mislead students intentionally.

A COUPLE OF FAKE SYNDROMES

I was supposed to present a case in the student conference the following week. Under the guise of a practical joke, one by one, I told each of the residents and the students, as well as our attending, that I would be presenting a couple of fictitious cases before I brought out the real one. No one knew who I told or who I was pranking, but they were a good-natured bunch and everyone was in on it. I never did, however, let Barry in on the joke. He had no idea of what I was planning.

On the day of the conference, I stood in front of the group and read from my notes. I looked around and I could see a twinkle in the occasional eye as I talked.

"The first case I am going to discuss is a rare condition known as Nuahcerpel Syndrome."

I paused and looked around the room. Barry was in the back and I could see his wheels were turning. I think he was actually trying to recall such a syndrome.

"Nuahcerpel Syndrome is an autosomal dominant genetic disorder which produces short stature, large ears, high voice, and extreme irritability. People with this disorder are short tempered and often get into fights with others. It is been found that they have aurophilia such that medicinal compounds containing inorganic gold will actually produce a state of euphoria."

Needless to say, "nuahcperel" was "leprechaun" spelled backwards. A couple of the students got it right away and I could hear an occasional chuckle. This seemed to puzzle Barry.

My attending was beaming as I continued.

"The second case is Alucard Syndrome, named after the first reported sufferer of this condition. It is generally believed to be autosomal recessive although there have been acquired cases reported. The key features of the disorder are tall stature, malformed teeth, photophobia, and severe anemia that requires frequent transfusions."

The group was loving it. Several people immediately caught on to the word "Dracula" being spelled backwards.

Barry still hadn't caught on, so I continued my deception.

I asked, "Would anyone like to comment on these two conditions? Has anyone seen a case of either one?"

I am a terrible person. I looked to the back of the room and addressed Barry, "Barry, what do you think about these disorders? Do you think there might be a common genetic thread?"

Barry looked around the room and began to speak. "I don't know about the first syndrome, but the second one sounds familiar. I think there was a paper about it in the *Journal of Hematology* a couple of years ago, but I would have to look in my records. These are fascinating cases and I'm very glad you brought them to our attention.

The room cracked up, and Barry didn't understand why they were all laughing. As things began to calm down, I presented my real case and we continued with the conference.

It wasn't until later that day that Barry figured out that I had set him up. He never talked to me again, and as far as I could tell, he wasn't quite so free with his wisdom to the other medical students. I often wonder what kind of pediatrician he turned out to be. He probably has a dartboard with my picture on it.

Lesson learned: Sometimes you need to deflate an ego.

DESPERATION AND A HACKSAW BLADE

It was very important for me to begin the neurosurgical rotation that I had set up the previous year. Just to give you an idea about how badly I wanted to be on the service, here is a little story.

About halfway through my previous rotation at Michael Reese, I was running across campus because I was late for rounds. Being blessed with clumsiness, I twisted my foot in a hole in front of the hospital. I went down like a bowling pin. Like most people who do something as stupid as that, I quickly looked around to be sure that no one saw me. Unfortunately, my clumsy act had a witness. As I sat there, one of the senior medical students saw me go down and hurried over.

"Ed, you okay?"

I gave him a look that gave justice to the stupidity of that question.

"I suppose so."

I tried to get to my feet, and when I put weight upon my left foot, my world almost ended. The pain was intense.

My friend helped me hobble into the emergency room that fortunately wasn't very far from where I fell.

One of the ER nurses who knew me noted us coming in through the sliding electric door. I was waiting for something funny from her sharp tongue.

"What the hell happened to you?" she almost sympathetically said. I must've looked like I was in a lot of pain.

As I was trying to come up with a clever answer, she shoved a wheelchair under me and wheeled me over to the main area. I waved a thank you to my friend, and I was soon lying on a gurney.

I looked at her and said with mustered up seriousness, "I think I just need an x-ray. Probably a sprain. I've done this before."

"Yeah, right. That foot looks mighty swollen."

The ER attending saw me and ordered an x-ray. When I was wheeled back to the ER, he told me that he was calling orthopedics.

"When did you break that foot the first time?"

"I didn't know it had broken before. One time, I was in a faraway and unfriendly place and I fell a good distance to the ground. It hurt for a while, but I didn't know it was broken at the time."

"Well, now you have two metatarsal fractures. The fresh one is more of an avulsion and the other one has healed a little bit deformed. You must've been walking on it after you broke it."

I did. At the time, I had no choice. I limped for quite a while after that event.

Before long, the orthopedics resident put me in a clunky plaster cast. My first concern was my upcoming neurosurgical rotation. I still had a few weeks before it started, but I knew that there was no way they would allow me in the operating room with a filthy plaster cast on my leg.

In medicine, it is very common for physicians to treat our patients better than we would treat ourselves. I hope that is always the case. I foolishly decided that I would lose the cast before I limped onto the Neurosurgery floor.

The night before the rotation was to begin, I bought a hack saw blade and sawed off the plaster cast. I gingerly put my weight down on the foot and it wasn't that painful. I decided that a little bit of pain was better than losing a fantastic neurosurgical rotation. I then became the owner of two poorly healed metatarsal fractures. Looking back, it was worth it.

NEUROSURGERY

Once I had completed my basic general rotations, I was eligible to sign up for a neurosurgical rotation, and I wanted to be with the best. I arranged to be on the service of Dr. Oscar Sugar, the Chairman of Neurosurgery at the University of Illinois. He was an international figure. Dr. Sugar was known for his historic surgical separation of Siamese twins joined at the head, and his pioneering work in pediatric Neurosurgery and Neurosurgery education. In all of my interactions with neurosurgeons both prior to that time and since that time, Dr. Sugar remains the most compassionate and gentle of all my teachers. He was a true gentleman and a brilliant surgeon.

I limped to my first day on the service, and fortunately, no one asked me what was wrong with my foot.

Dr. Sugar's service was well run and his surgeons respected him. People knew they had to do their jobs, but they never felt threatened. It was one of those rare situations where people were truly inspired to do a good job. As a result, he produced some very fine surgeons.

I remember my first day on his service. He introduced himself and told me that he expected a lot from his students. He would make rounds with me and the senior Neurosurgery resident each day, and he told me that I needed to be up-to-date on reading about these patients at all times. He didn't have to tell me twice.

For some reason, and others have noted the same thing, you *wanted* to do a good job because his approval was so important. I've never met anyone else like that in my life. I'm generally not an approval seeker, and that particular character flaw has gotten me into trouble in other settings. This was different.

The senior neurosurgical resident, we will call Dr. Dean Howard, seemed like a good guy — very intense — and seemed like a person who didn't take crap from anyone.

JUDY THE CHEERLEADER

We started rounds and came to the first room. As we stood outside the door, Howard summarized the case. The patient was a 16-year-old high school cheerleader; we will call her Judy, who had been jumping on a trampoline. She fell off the trampoline, landed on her head, and broke her neck in the high cervical region. This made her quadriplegic (paralyzed in all four extremities), but she could still breathe on her own. When she arrived at the University of Illinois Hospital, Dr. Sugar operated almost immediately to stabilize the broken bones in her neck. She had only been awake for a few hours, as they had cut back on her strong pain medications. No movement was noted post op. She was probably going to remain paralyzed.

Howard had the chart, and he reviewed the latest vital signs and laboratory data. Judy would be on our service for a few more days until she was properly stabilized, and then she would be sent to a large rehab facility in downtown Chicago.

We walked into the room to see her on what is called a Stryker frame, a device that looks like a narrow canvas stretcher underneath the patient, with fixtures to place another stretcher on top, like a sandwich. Large stainless steel wheels allow the apparatus to turn the patient over. The purpose was to distribute pressure and avoid bedsores, but a good part of the time, the patient was facing the floor, looking down through a hole in the upper stretcher. It looked like something from the Spanish Inquisition.

When we came into the room, we saw Judy lying on her back and crying quietly. She was able to move her face but her arms and legs were flaccid. We stood for a moment, watching her and waiting for her to notice us. She was a pretty high school girl who was probably very popular... Now she was totally paralyzed, and the reality was beginning to sink in.

Dr. Sugar approached the bed and put his hand on her arm. She stopped crying and looked at him expectantly. He took a paper tissue from the bedside table and dabbed her eyes and her nose. She smiled at him through her tears.

"Judy, my name is Doctor Sugar. The last time I saw you, you were asleep in the operating room. Do you have any pain?"

His calm grandfatherly way brought her a smile as she told him, "Just a little. Doctor, when will I be able to start moving my arms and legs?"

He pulled up a chair and sat next to her and we stood back. He looked at her sadly and said, "Judy, I don't know if you ever will. You had a severe injury to your spinal cord, and it's just too early to tell what muscle function you might recover."

Judy began sobbing. "Why does it have to happen to me?"

He looked at her and smiled, again dabbing away her tears. "We stabilized the fracture in your neck. That's why you were in the operating room last night. Your spinal cord was damaged from that fall. At this point, the only thing you can do is pray, and we will do our best to take good care of you."

It was a moving moment, and even Howard's tough exterior looked a little misty.

As we left the room we could hear little Judy crying behind us. It was bitter crying with sobs. It was the kind of uncontrollable crying that accompanies a great loss.

THE ANEURYSM

The Neurosurgery service dealt with emergencies such as Judy's as well as elective, scheduled cases. Dr. Sugar had cases referred to him from great distances because of his reputation.

An hour later, we were heading for the operating room for a scheduled aneurysm repair. An aneurysm is an enlargement of an artery. When this occurs near the brain, it can be very dangerous. A cerebral aneurysm can rupture and produce instant death.

The patient who was about to be operated upon had an aneurysm of the left posterior communicating artery. Because an aneurysm in this location can press on nerve fibers leading to the pupil, the diagnosis was suspected when he developed an enlarged pupil. Testing was done to establish the diagnosis. It was relatively lucky for the patient. The best luck is not to have an aneurysm; the next best is to find it before it bursts.

The location was dangerous because it was somewhat difficult to get to. If any leaking or bleeding takes place, the patient could lose his ability to speak and understand, if they even survived the bleed. Because of the difficulty of the case, another one of the attendings was going to assist, with Dr. Howard as a second assistant and me as a useless observer. This type of operation was the surgical equivalent of a bomb squad defusing a bomb.

I squinted from a distance to watch the procedure as they made a horseshoe-shaped incision in the scalp and pulled back the soft tissue. Next, they drilled four holes in the skull. Using a saw, they connected the holes and lifted a flap of bone, like a trap door. From where I was standing, I could see the brain pulsate. Next, they sliced into the dura, which is the leathery membrane that surrounds the brain. From then on, I couldn't see very much.

Dr. Sugar essentially narrated his work as they eventually reached in and carefully placed a clip on the neck of the aneurysm, preventing any further threat of bleeding. This aneurysm was like a cherry on a stem, so they crimped a metal clip on the stem to stop any further blood flow to that weakened area. It seemed to take forever to get that far...and just as long for them to retrace their steps until the final scalp stitch. Hours had passed, but my legs didn't even feel tired. I was totally fascinated. It was amazing!

It was then that an interesting thing happened. Dr. Sugar went up to his office and literally typed his entire report. His fingers flew on the keys of the old typewriter. He explained to me that it was easier to do it this way, rather than to dictate, read, make corrections, etcetera. He probably could type a lot faster than his secretary could.

While he was typing, the other neurosurgical attending was busy wielding colored pencils to sketch the procedure. He was a gifted artist and he skillfully created a reproduction of the aneurysm, not unlike the famous medical illustrations of Dr. Frank Netter. Of course, they could've taken photographs, but they didn't. The charts from that service were like textbooks. We could look through the charts and learn... unlike the sloppy computer-generated records that we see in hospitals today.

Lesson learned: Neurosurgery requires extreme mental discipline.

NEUROSURGERY CALL

The neurosurgical call schedule was just as brutal as it was on general surgery. I was assigned to Howard, and we were on call every other night. We had a general surgery intern as well, but Howard didn't want to delegate anything to a non-neurosurgeon. Howard said he was "just unskilled labor, putting in his time."

One day, at the end of the afternoon, one of the Neurosurgery attendings told us to go get supper; he would cover the house as long as we left the general surgery rotating intern behind to do the scutwork.

Howard and I had the same idea; we turned to each other and said "The Greeks." We walked double-time over to The Greeks and went directly into the Monkey Room. We got a corner table and sat with our backs to the wall. We got a chance to talk.

Howard was about my age, but he started medical school only two years late. He had a two-year diversion to the Republic of South Vietnam as a draftee. We compared stories and resisted the temptation to have a beer, which usually has to accompany such stories. We connected well.

As we ate, one of the surgical residents from County walked quickly into the Monkey Room, looked around, and came right up to us.

"Dr. Howard, I understand you guys are covering neurosurg for County tonight, right?"

Howard looked at him and said, "Yeah... so?"

"We have a multiple trauma who didn't wake up... We sutured his leg and set his fracture...."

Howard was pissed. "Don't you think the brain is more important than that other shit?"

The guy from County didn't know what to say. He looked at me and I shrugged. What the hell did I know?

Howard was up, throwing money on the table for both our partially eaten meals, and we set off for the familiar County ER.

The surgery resident led us into one of the ER side rooms. A 30-ish black man was laying there, a cast on his right leg and bandage covering his left hand. The man was breathing regularly, but did not respond to us yelling at him or pinching him. Howard shined a light in each eye.

"He hasn't blown a pupil yet, but look at the raccoon eyes. He at least has a basilar skull fracture. Look at the bruising behind his ears..."

The man had two shiners, and had blood coming from his right ear canal. Howard went over to the x-ray screen and looked at the skull and neck x-rays.

"At least we know he didn't have a cervical fracture and...." He paused, and then pointed to the front view of the skull. "Look at this! His falx is being pushed to the left!"

As I said earlier, we didn't yet have CT scanning available, so we resorted to the tools at hand. A plain x-ray can sometimes show calcification of the falx cerebri. This structure separates the halves of the brain. If you think of the brain as a walnut with two halves, the falx is the membrane that separates the two. This frequently is calcified so it is visible in plain x-rays. It's supposed to be in the midline, so if it's off center, there is probably a mass pushing it.... Like a hemorrhage.

Howard turned to me, excited at the prospect of a surgical case. "This guy has a right frontal subdural. We've got to take him to surgery right now. If there is no family to sign a consent, we'll declare it an emergency."

He grabbed a surgical prep kit from a shelf in the trauma room and shaved the entire front half patient's head, saying, "This guy needed a haircut anyway."

It seemed like moments later when Howard and I were scrubbing at the sink in front of the operating room at County. I could see the anesthesiologist with his colorful surgical cap preparing to put the patient to sleep. He raised both thumbs and smiled at us. Not that the patient wasn't already asleep, but you need to seriously anesthetize a guy when you're going to drill a hole in his head.

Howard based his decision on his clinical evaluation and a simple x-ray; he knew that there had to be a big blood clot pressing on the right side of the brain. We now depend on CT scans or MRIs, but there is still no substitute for clinical judgment.

He continued his teaching while we scrubbed. "Since there was no fracture in that area, it must have been a blunt trauma. What if there had been a fracture line in the right temple?"

"I guess we would need to worry about epidural hematoma, right?"

He smiled. "Right on."

A subdural hematoma is a collection of blood that accumulates below the dura, the leathery lining around the brain. It's usually due to a traumatic brain injury that results in tearing the veins that bridge the gap between the dura and the surface of the brain. This has the potential of compressing the brain, raising pressure in the head, and potentially causing death.

An epidural hematoma is due to a fracture of the skull that has torn the blood vessels inside the skull. Blood accumulates outside of the dura, still producing compression of the brain. It is also quite dangerous and can be fatal.

We finished scrubbing under the watchful eye of the OR nurse. I swear they are all the same. Very protective.

The patient was positioned on his back, his head turned to the left, positioned with rolled up towels and tape. Howard turned to me and said, "This is how we prep the scalp."

He proceeded to scrub the man's shaved head with sponge sticks soaked in an antiseptic solution. He drew ever-increasing circles from where his incision was going to be. He did this several times, throwing away the sponge stick with each step.

Howard then took a scalpel and made an incision about where he expected the subdural hematoma to be. He cut clean and deep, in a U-shaped form, and peeled back the scalp and other tissues to expose the bone of the skull. It took a few minutes to control the bleeding from the scalp and the underlying tissues. He showed me how to grip the edge of the wound with gauze and apply pressure while he worked with the electrocautery to zap bleeding vessels.

Next, he took a hand drill and began boring into the skull. It sounds quite barbaric, but this was a life-saving procedure. He drilled an opening about the size of a nickel, exposing the dura.

"This membrane looks pretty tense. Definitely a subdural."

He made an incision in the dura, and blood welled up. He carefully suctioned out the blood as it poured out of the incision. It hadn't fully clotted yet. When he felt he had cleaned out the remaining blood, it was time to close the wound.

"Ever stitch before?"

I told him about my time at County and general surgery. He nodded and began to close the dura and then the deep tissue over the burr hole.

"Okay, Messina, now you can close the scalp."

I proceeded to use absorbable suture material in the deep thick layers beneath the skin as Howard nodded his approval. Then, I used black suture silk to close the skin — a true work of art. I took my time and spaced the sutures perfectly, a totally useless thing to do. It doesn't really matter how pretty the skin sutures are, but it was a matter of pride and craftsmanship.

The patient was sent to recovery while we cleaned up. We went back to The Greeks to try again to eat something. We called back to our service, and the attending was still there catching up on paperwork, so he told us to take our time. He knew that we had just dealt with that subdural.

It's a good feeling to know that you have made a big difference in somebody's life. We ate ravenously and then we walked back to the recovery room.

We found our patient awake and looking around the room. We also noticed that his arm was cuffed to the gurney and a cop was standing nearby.

The cop told us that our patient had jumped out of the window at a crime scene after beating a woman senseless. The reason we didn't see his victim was because she died on the way to the hospital.

"Well Doc, looks like you saved the wrong one."

It wasn't our choice to make.

Lesson learned: It doesn't matter who the patient is, we are doctors, and they are the patients.

The Neurosurgery rotation was wonderful. At the end of the rotation, Dr. Sugar invited me to his office to have a chat. He told me that he was going to write a good evaluation for me, and he knew that Dr. Howard was going to do the same. He asked me what my interests were for the future.

"Well, I really like Neurosurgery and I like Neurology. I feel that I need to narrow it down further, but I would also like to deepen my understanding in both fields."

He looked at me, saying, "You're in the James Scholar program, right?"

I nodded.

"Well, it would serve you very well if you spent some time in neuropathology and neuroradiology. They may help narrow things down. If you've got the time, I can recommend you to spend time with Dr. Orville Bailey for a while."

Dr. Bailey was one of the most famous neuropathologists in the world, and his labs were only a couple of floors above where we were talking. This particular neuropathology rotation was a tremendous opportunity, and it was only available to students who have been recommended for it. I jumped at the chance and made an appointment to talk to him.

I was already scheduled for another basic rotation, but Dr. Bailey said that I could start with him as soon as it was over.

DR. ORVILLE BAILEY

The white-haired Dr. Bailey was one of the originators of the field of neuropathology, and his books were widely published. He allowed one student at a time to rotate with him, and I was incredibly fortunate to be selected, thanks to Dr. Sugar.

Neuropathology is the study of diseases of the nervous system. The very basis of neurologic disease is defined by slicing brains taken from autopsies and by examining the tissue under the microscope – all done by a neuropathologist.

Dr. Bailey guided me on which books to read, each dealing specifically with the classification of brain tumors. He led me to a small cove in his laboratory, which contained a single table with a microscope. The walls were covered with shelves. On the shelves were countless boxes of microscope slides.

He told me that some of the slides were irreplaceable, and these slides must not be removed from that room. He also told me that under no circumstances should I drop or break any slides by rolling the microscope down too low. As time passed, I noticed that many of the slides had handwritten labels. Many of these specimens were actually prepared by famous scientists such as Santiago Ramon y Cajal. I was surprised that he allowed a mere medical student to handle these historic pieces of work.

I came to the lab promptly at 8:00 AM each day, my head full of what I'd read the night before about brain tumor anatomy and histology. This material was much more detailed than what I had studied in general pathology. Dr. Bailey would discuss different tumors with me, sometimes taking me to another room where he had jars of brains and parts of brains to show me what the tumors looked like before they went under the microscope.

He told me which slides I should look at, and I made copious notes as I worked. What I learned in Dr. Bailey's lab remained useful to me when I took my Neurology specialty boards many years later. This was classic neuropathology, the basis of Neurology and Neurosurgery.

THE BRAIN CUTTING

Every week Dr. Bailey would preside over the brain cutting at Cook County Hospital. Brain cutting is a tradition among neurologists, neurosurgeons, neuropathologists, and neuroradiologists.

When the brain is removed fresh from an autopsy, it has the consistency of firm gelatin. It deteriorates very rapidly unless it is properly preserved. Autopsy brains are soaked in a solution of formalin for a couple of weeks in order to fix the tissue. These firmed-up brains are then sliced in order to understand the cause of death of their former owners.

On brain cutting day, the elderly Dr. Bailey, his equally elderly secretary, and I walked a couple of blocks in a slow parade to Cook County Hospital. The brain cuttings were held in an old-fashioned surgical amphitheater with steep seating. The sessions were usually attended by the neurological and neurosurgical staff of the University of Illinois, Cook County Hospital, Rush medical Center, and others from across town.

When we first entered the amphitheater, I looked up to see many faces watching us make our way to the bottom row of seats. It looked like paintings I had seen from late 19th century Paris when Dr. Jean Martin Charcot established the discipline of Neurology... mainly through brain cutting. Every eye was watching Dr. Bailey.

Dr. Bailey was very traditional. He did not use a Dictaphone. Instead, his elderly secretary took shorthand as he described his findings. He was also a stickler for having a clean, properly starched white coat and a pair of clean, old-fashioned rubber gloves waiting for him. His secretary dusted talc inside the gloves before he put them on.

The usual protocol was for the physician who cared for the deceased patient to present a brief clinical summary. This usually was the job of an intern or resident. It was not for the faint hearted, since they were essentially telling the story of one of their patients who had died.

In medicine, it does not matter *why* someone dies; we still think of it as a personal failure. It's part of the collective physician ego.

The first case was being presented by a Neurology resident from Rush Medical Center, which was down the street. I honestly did not listen to the history or examination. I was completely entranced by the four brains lined up on the dissection table.

These were *actual brains*, cut from recently deceased persons, containing, up until the moment of their death, the entire story of their life. The brain, which learned, loved, and hated. The brain that caused actions and reactions, and caused the person to be who they were. Death and a formalin solution made these marvelous organs into firm, congealed, lifeless objects. We would learn from these objects. These brains were different from the ones in the anatomy lab. These brains had a story behind them.

When the resident, whom I was ignoring, was finished with his presentation, a neuroradiologist stood up while his crew was wheeling in a large portable screen, which was then plugged in. He walked over and began slapping x-ray films onto it. He spoke the entire time, pointing out abnormalities on the arteriograms and plain x-ray films. A year later when I was on the neuroradiology service, we were showing people CT scan films on this same view box. A new era began as quickly as that. Today, it's PowerPoint and MRI and PET scan images.

When the presentations and the x-ray discussion were finished, all eyes went to Dr. Bailey. He got up from his place in the lowest row of seats and walked over to the dissecting table. His secretary was right behind him, steno pad at the ready.

Dr. Bailey looked up at the group and slid the brain of the first patient to the middle of the table. He spoke loudly and with authority.

"The cortical surface of the brain is well developed with mild atrophy, age-appropriate."

He held it up for everyone to see. It was pale because it had been soaking in the fixative. He stated that the gyri (or hills) of the brain were flattened.

He turned up the brain so that the bottom could be seen by all. The part of the brain known as the uncus, on the right side, was bulging out next to the brain stem.

"This appears to be uncal herniation, brought about by mass effect."

He was showing us a deformity of the brain caused by brain swelling, which pushed the brain downward. This had subsequently compressed the brain stem, causing the patient to die of respiratory arrest and cardiovascular collapse.

"Now we will look for the cause of the increased intracranial pressure."

He made a single slice across the brain and held it up for everyone to see. There was a huge hemorrhage on the right side of the brain. There was murmuring among the crowd. Apparently, some had predicted this.

"This looks like a classic hypertensive hemorrhage." He said.

Dr. Bailey continued the brain cutting, selecting various parts of the brain and dropping them into a jar of liquid. These would later be put into paraffin so they could be thinly sliced and placed under the microscope. Perhaps some of those slides would be added to the slide room in his lab.

This was indeed the final diagnosis, the incontrovertible explanation for why the patient died.

Nowadays, we use CT or MR scanning to show us these abnormalities during life, so the brain cutting is usually less surprising. It is nevertheless a critical part of medical education.

The drama of the amphitheater, the formality of the case presentations, and the quiet competence of Dr. Bailey will always live in my mind. I've been to many brain cuttings in my career, but these first days remain vivid to me.

BROWN GRAVY

I made it a point to avoid pediatrics at Cook County Hospital, because there was a chance that I could be assigned to a floor called The Diarrhea Ward. This was a service where kids were kept in isolation, and they were there to be rehydrated. Medical students invariably caught diarrhea from these kids. To me, it didn't sound like a very good way to learn medicine.

Diarrhea unfortunately entered my life when I was on the Infectious Disease service with Dr. George Gee Jackson. It's not that I caught the illness, but I was part of the team that would track it down, as an exercise in epidemiology.

The Infectious Disease service dealt with communicable diseases ranging from malaria to tuberculosis and other disorders. Although Dr. Jackson was an international figure in his field, he still felt it was appropriate for our service to help track down a recent minor outbreak of diarrhea among medical students and nurses.

In reality, it was actually a very educational experience. The Infectious Disease fellow was in charge of the quest. An infectious disease fellow — or ID fellow — is a physician who has completed Internal Medicine training and then spends a couple of years concentrating on the diagnosis and treatment of infectious diseases.

Our fellow told us that we needed to interview people who had caught diarrhea within the past few days and create a grid to see what they had in common.

We interviewed the different shifts of nurses at the University of Illinois Hospital, we checked with the medical students who were on service within the last few days, and we talked to everyone else who said they had had diarrhea within the last few days. I must say, it was sort of weird asking perfect strangers who were walking across campus whether they recently had diarrhea. I got the strangest looks from people, not to mention some interesting sarcastic responses.

We created a grid that listed all the people and all the places they had been, and we finally tracked down the culprit. What they had in common was the hospital cafeteria. The next step was to figure out what they had eaten. Ultimately, we discovered it was the brown gravy, lending it to the obvious jokes.

As trivial as this sounds, this was the same technique we might have used to explore an outbreak of a catastrophic communicable disease in a larger population. I learned a valuable technique, but I also learned to keep away from the brown gravy in the future.

THE VA HOSPITAL AND PROBLEMS WITH HEAT AND TEMPERATURES

It was a warm spring day and I was still on the Infectious Disease service. My job was to go over to one of the floors at the VA and check the temperature chart on a patient we had been seeing for an unidentified fever.

A fever of unknown origin (FUO) in adults is defined as a temperature higher than 100.9°F that lasts more than three weeks and has no obvious source. These are often very difficult to diagnose, so they consulted the Infectious Disease service.

I was already sweating as I walked two blocks from the University Hospital to the Westside VA hospital. I was enjoying the hot sun as I thought about the differential diagnosis of FUO. As I looked up at the hospital, I noticed that many of the windows were open, which seemed normal on a warm day such as that, although I wondered why they were not using the air-conditioning.

When I got to the floor, I noticed that the heat was on full tilt. I could feel it coming through the heating system, but the windows were wide open. It turned out that they were trying to use up their heating allowance so they wouldn't have a reduced heating budget the following year. One of my residents told me that this was typical in the VA system. Government logic, bureaucratic manipulation, and taxpayers' dollars. Indeed!

The rooms were not uncomfortable even though the heat was on because of the open windows and the fans that were running. I found the chart of the patient I was going to evaluate, and I noticed there were no temperatures written on it.

The temperature chart can show fluctuations in temperature that may have diagnostic significance. Fevers have different behaviors, and it's important to see when they spike and when they come down.

I asked one of the nurses where the temperatures were, and she pointed to the temperature clipboard. I went to the board and found that there were no temperatures recorded for the past six hours in this patient with fever. When I asked her what was going on, she just shrugged and walked away.

FOLEY MAGIC

When I got to the ward where the patient with the fever was waiting for me, I ran into one of my friends from a previous rotation.

"Hey, Chuck. What's happening?" He was dressed in surgical scrubs, and he didn't look happy.

"I had to leave the damned OR because some guy is bleeding all over his bed on the ward."

I was already on his ward, so I walked with him, hoping it wasn't the patient I was looking for.

A few beds down, I could see a large red stain on the sheets of an old vet's bed. The nurse was standing there, looking furious. She handed Chuck a Foley catheter.

"Here. He's your problem now. He's so demented that he doesn't even know what he did."

A Foley catheter is a tube that you thread through the urethra into the bladder so urine can flow. It's used on people who have obstructions or people who are incontinent. It is really two tubes together; one is the tube that drains the bladder and the other is attached to a balloon at the end, which is inflated with sterile water to prevent the catheter from sliding out.

The nurse had handed Chuck a bloody Foley catheter that was still inflated.

"Chuck," I said, incredulously, "he pulled out an inflated Foley! How the hell did he get it through his urethra?"

"No shit. I guess that explains the blood. Right Sherlock? He did this last week also. Had to call Urology because he tore his urethra when he yanked it out. They're gonna love this."

Chuck was showing the classic signs of burnout. It happens to overworked students and house-staff when they see that all their efforts achieve nothing.

I'm hoping that the VA system has improved since 37 years ago. At the time, it was my first taste of what socialized medicine might be like. I frankly was not used to this nonsense, because I was exposed to such excellent nursing at the University of Illinois Hospital and Michael Reese, as well as Cook County Hospital.

I'M GLAD IT'S NOT MY BRAIN

CT scanning first came to Chicago when I was in medical school. The technology originally was developed in England in the early 1970s. When these machines first came to America, we originally called them EMI scanners. EMI stood for *Electronic Musical Instruments*, and I believe they also had the contract for the Beatles at that time. They later were called CT scans.

The first EMI scans were somewhat crude, but they were worlds better than the classical radioactive brain scans that we were used to. The image was at first only a couple hundred pixels in either direction. Currently they are more like 1024 x 1024. The patient's head was placed into a type of skullcap that looked like a giant condom, and I believe water circulated outside of this rubber barrier to keep the heat down.

This was a huge step in medicine, especially in neurology. We were then able to see the living brain and even be able to see a brain tumor if it was big enough. It changed everything. I remember my classmates telling me that it was foolish for me to become a neurologist because my job would be replaced by the CT scanner. Ha!

I remember sitting in the control room with one of my instructors, watching the tiny black and white screen that showed the brain image. It was very slow, but we were in awe of the technology. Up until then, all images in medicine were visible only on x-ray film. This was digital, although we had no idea what that term would later come to mean.

We sat at the scanner watching the images gradually come onto the screen. The scan had been done earlier, and the computer was showing each image in sequence as it processed it, as if the brain had been sliced horizontally about every half-inch. It was similar to the way a brain is sectioned in a brain cutting. Having spent time with Dr. Bailey, I had a pretty good feel for external brain anatomy. The brain in the picture looked somewhat shriveled up. We call this atrophy.

Trying to seem knowledgeable, I piped up, "Wow, look at that atrophy. I'm glad that's not my brain."

My instructor looked at me, hesitated a moment, and then said with no expression, "Well, it's *my* brain. We used me as a test subject."

He waited for my reaction. I honestly didn't know what to say. I looked at the image and saw his name typed at the bottom of each picture.

Lesson learned: Be sure you know whose brain image you are looking at before you blurt out a comment.

NEUROLOGY OR NEUROSURGERY?

A difficult choice for a medical student is deciding which specialty to go into. Students often make this choice because of exposure to good role models. In recent years, medical students have been conditioned, if not pressured, to go into primary care from early in medical school. This may explain some of the apathy that I have noticed in some young doctors who later regret that choice.

Medicine is all about passion. This is a driving force to excel in one's chosen field and tolerate the rigorous training for so many years. If a doctor does not absolutely love what they are doing, they are doing themselves and their patients a disservice. Patients can tell. I hear it all the time from people telling me why they are changing primary physicians.

By the end of my third year in medical school, I was quite certain that I was going to become either a neurologist or a neurosurgeon. The problem was that I couldn't make up my mind which one to choose. I returned for another neurology rotation at Michael Reese to help me decide.

At the end of that neurology rotation, I sat down with Dr. Klawans to discuss my career direction. He was supportive of me choosing neurology; in fact, he offered me a position in his residency program. He understood, however, that I was looking for a larger program to launch a future academic career. He told me that he would write me a personal letter of recommendation to whichever chairperson I chose.

I likewise met with Dr. Sugar. He also offered me a position in his neurosurgical residency program, but told me he would gladly write a personal letter to any neurosurgery chairperson I chose.

I began making applications to both neurology and neurosurgical programs. I could not make up my mind. In those days, neurology and neurosurgical residencies did not use the National Residency Matching Program that's used today. You basically had to make individual deals with different programs, holding out for the ones you wanted the most.

Internal Medicine and general surgery programs used the Match so I needed to make a choice because these were necessary prerequisites for the residencies I would be choosing. I had to match with an Internal Medicine internship if I chose neurology, or I had to match with at least two years of general surgery if I chose neurosurgery.

The problem was that I was still unable to make up my mind. I was receiving requests for interviews from neurology and neurosurgical programs. I interviewed at some very impressive places like Washington

University and Johns Hopkins, Baylor, Mayo, Yale, and many others. In the weeks that followed, I was getting acceptance letters to both neurology and neurosurgical programs at the better teaching hospitals.

I still could not make up my mind!

One day, getting out of bed bleary-eyed from only three hours of sleep, I almost tripped over my dog, Guinevere. I realized that even a minor injury, like a sprained hand (or another broken foot), would keep me from doing neurosurgery for weeks at a time.

I was also considering the fact that I was graduating from medical school at almost 31 years of age. I was concerned that someday I might have to halt my neurosurgical career if I developed any physical problems or became less coordinated. As a neurologist, I reasoned, I could work much later in life and still work with the beloved brain. In retrospect, I am more than certain I made the right choice.

This was how I made up my mind. Blame it on the dog. I ended up accepting the neurology residency position at Washington University in St. Louis at Barnes Hospital. It has historically been among the best hospitals in the country, and it still is. I was thrilled to be accepted into the Department of Neurology under Dr. William Landau. The department had the faculty, prestige, and visibility to launch my career. To this day, I am proud to say I was trained there.

MY PRESUMPTUOUS VERSION OF THE "MODEL OF THE MIND"

This is not about me as much as it describes the naive presumptuousness of a senior medical student.

I still had some elective time left before graduation, so I indulged myself in the joys of purely selfish research. I didn't know enough to know that I didn't know enough. As Frank Capra said in his book, *The Name Above the Title*, people in their 20s can do great things because they don't know what is being called impossible by older people.

I had some thoughts about how the brain must function...It was a theory about neuronal function and I am still working on it to this day. This remains the holy grail of neuroscience.

I had an idea that it would be possible to influence certain brain functions, including behavior, if we knew how to reach them physiologically and modify them with guided stimuli.

I presented some of my neophyte theories to Dr. Klawans, and he suggested I discuss these with Dr. Roy R. Grinker Sr., who was a giant in the field of biological psychiatry. He authored many seminal works dealing with personality disorders, schizophrenia, and depression.

Dr. Grinker had written the well-known textbook, *Grinker's Neurology*, and had coined the term "battle fatigue" (now called PTSD) during World War II. He was the last living student of Sigmund Freud, but he was a strong proponent of the biopsychosocial approach to understanding human behavior. It seemed logical for me to talk to him.

I needed a way to approach this great man. It dawned on me that I needed to create a graphic representation of my hypothesis of how the brain worked, because I couldn't describe it properly with words. I bought a roll of white shelf paper and cut two, three-foot lengths, which I taped side by side, forming one huge piece of paper.

I started writing in pencil, needless to say, creating a flow chart of my theory of brain functions, leaving a large empty space for "personality."

I got an appointment with Dr. Grinker at his office at the Psychosomatic and Psychiatric Institute (P&PI) at Michael Reese. I was very nervous to present what might seem like drivel to this man as I sat in the waiting room at the P&PI.

After what seemed an eternity (but actually exactly at the time of our scheduled meeting), he came out and invited me into his office, large paper roll and all. I unrolled it on a table and began to explain my hypotheses.

Dr. Grinker listened politely and asked questions as he pointed to different parts of my diagram. We kept coming back to the blank area for "personality." When I left his office, I knew I needed to beef up my concept of personality as it applied to brain physiology. Needless to say, this was extremely presumptuous of me.

To help fill in this gap, I was fortunate enough to meet with Dr. Theodore Millon, who was head psychologist at the Neuropsychiatric Institute at the University of Illinois at that time. He is still the guru of personality theory. He also patiently listened to my ideas and asked many good questions.

The main thing I learned after spending time with these giants was that I needed a better way to explain the complexity of the brain with its countless pathways and trillions of connections. Again, this sounds presumptuous and audacious now, but I was very serious at the time. Time flew by and I put the project on hold when my Internal Medicine internship was to begin.

After all this time, I have not abandoned these early thoughts. In recent years, I have developed and patented an artificial intelligence language called FloBase® that may be a helpful tool in expressing these youthful thoughts. The show's not over yet.

Lesson learned: When you have what you think is a worthwhile idea, look for the smartest people you can find so you can talk about it. Other people might not understand.

MEDICAL SCHOOL IN RETROSPECT

Once I had been accepted into a neurology residency, which would begin about two years later, I still had my final year in medical school to complete.

I had pretty much completed all my required rotations, and I completed all my year-end clinical exams. I continued doing elective rotations that would best prepare me for Internal Medicine and Neurology.

I spent many weeks at Rush for neuroradiology under Dr. Michael Huckman. I continued to return to Michael Reese for other rotations.

I had a wonderful experience in hematology with Dr. Margaret Telfer and Dr. Mabel Koshy. My final rotation at Michael Reese was the ER. I figured it would prepare me the best for what lay ahead. By now, the nurses had gotten used to me and actually trusted me... for a medical student, at least.

MATCH DAY

I needed to do at least a one-year internship in Internal Medicine before my residency in St. Louis could begin. I made the program at Michael Reese my first choice on the National Residency Matching Program. If only Dr. Louis Sherwood would pick me on the Match, I would be a truly happy camper.

Although I knew Dr. Sherwood and most of the attendings on the residency selection committee, nothing was guaranteed. I knew that my future intern class had 28 first-year openings and that about 800 people had applied. I had some good second choices on my list, and the Neurology department at Washington University would somehow get me a spot in the medicine program — but I wanted to be at Michael Reese. At the time, I had no idea how it would change my life...

The day of the Match had come. In those days, a piece of paper was posted in one of the lecture halls at the Medical School. I mulled around and paced with my fellow medical students. We had all been driving ourselves crazy. Suddenly, one of the Dean's assistants entered the room and posted several sheets of paper on a wall in the front of the room. She literally ran to the back of the room to avoid being trampled, but she stuck around to witness the human drama.

Some people were shrieking with delight and others walked quietly away, with wistful half smiles. I was getting closer to the front of the crowd when a buddy of mine yelled from the front of the line, "Hey, Messina! We're both gonna be at Reese!"

I was overjoyed, but I still needed to see my name on that list. It was reminiscent of the day I got the letter of acceptance into medical school from Dr. Cerchio. I must have read it a hundred times.

I finally got close enough to see my name. Sure enough, it said "Michael Reese."

I was overjoyed that they matched me! It was my original dream before I even started medical school. I had no idea that it would prove to be the best and the toughest year of my life to date.

FINISHING UP MEDICAL SCHOOL IN THE ER

My final medical school rotation was in the Michael Reese emergency room again. I loved that emergency room because there was no end to the variety of problems that needed to be solved. I loved the adrenaline rushes. Granted, I hadn't been there for very long, but I thought I had seen most everything. Not by a long shot.

ICE CUBES IN THE JOCKEY SHORTS

Late one afternoon, the paramedics rushed a gurney past the sliding glass ER doors. One of them was bagging the patient.

He shouted, "Respiratory arrest" as they ran by.

The respiratory therapist ran over and took over, squeezing the Ambu bag. The rest of us lifted the bottom sheet off the stretcher and slid the man onto our hospital gurney.

The paramedic was out if breath as he said, "Probable junkie, found him on the street next to a pay phone. His friends probably called it in and ran. He also looks a little beaten up."

As my intern was intubating the man, that is, placing a tube down his trachea to breathe for him, the nurses started cutting off his clothing. Nurses with scissors can strip a patient's clothes off faster than a piranha can strip the meat off your bones. They stripped him because he might have been the victim of multiple trauma.

I was startled by the appearance of dozens of ice cubes clattering to the floor as they cut his underwear off. It briefly distracted me from placing an IV in his arm.

I went back to my task, but I couldn't help but ask, "What's with the ice cubes?"

The nurses said, "The junkies think that if they pack their nuts in ice, it'll wake them up from an overdose."

"Get out." I figured they were leading me on, like an initiation or something.

"No, seriously" she said, "when a junkie looks like he's going too far with an OD, his friends will pack his jockey shorts with ice cubes. That's probably what happened here."

My resident interrupted her. "Give him the Narcan."

Narcan, or naloxone, antagonizes the effect of opiates. Drugs that are related to opium such as heroine can be reversed by this drug. Overdoses of narcotics will suppress breathing, so this drug can be life saving when it reverses that effect.

The nurse pushed the drug into the IV that I had just started, along with some D50, which is a glucose solution. In about one or two minutes, the patient started moving around and moaning. He tried to pull out his IV as he started struggling.

Now that things were coming under control, my resident turned to me and said, "Don't be fooled by this guy waking up so quickly. Narcan doesn't last very long and we might need to repeat the dose based on how much heroine he actually took."

A few minutes later as we were discussing his case, the nurse walked over and said, "This guy wants to go home now. A real genius."

My resident looked up as if this happened all the time. "Well, tell him he can't. Besides, you cut up all his clothes."

"Yeah, he's pissed about that too."

"Tell him he has to stay."

She walked back to the bay and my resident turned to me again, saying, "The problem is that when you give them Narcan, it's almost like going into withdrawal. They get very antsy. It drives them crazy and they want to use again as soon as possible. The heroin effect might last longer than the Narcan, so we need to watch him. He could stop breathing again."

These days, cops and paramedics can give Narcan in the field, which makes things a lot simpler. It gives the ER a head start.

The nurse came back again. "His friends are in the waiting room and they have his long winter coat. He's gonna sign out AMA."

Signing out AMA means "against medical advice," and there's nothing we can do about it.

The resident looked exasperated, throwing down his pen. "Let me talk to him."

We walked back to the gurney. The patient was sitting on the edge, swearing up a storm, holding his sheets around him.

The resident eased him down onto his back again. "Listen, sir, you had a bad drug overdose and the medicine we just gave you is gonna wear off very soon. You're gonna start slipping away again, maybe stop breathing again."

"Bullshit. Where's my clothes? I'm gettin' outta here and you can't stop me. Is my woman in the waiting room?"

We walked away from him as the nurse was handing his overcoat to him.

"This guy is gonna look like a pervert when he gets back on the street wearing nothing but an overcoat and shoes."

The resident chuckled. "Yeah, but he's gonna slip away again. Oh well, we tried."

The addict signed himself out against medical advice. If he had stopped breathing again and died, we never heard about it.

OIL IN THE EAR

A 10-year-old kid came into the emergency room with his mom. He was screaming his lungs out and pawing at his right ear. His mom was trying to keep his hand from touching the ear. He was frantically clawing at the ear. By now, I had seen a few ear infections. They didn't act like this.

The nurses brought him into the pediatric examining area, and since things were slow on the adult side, I went in with the pediatric resident.

The boy was crying and screaming that his ear hurt. You would think that someone was dropping hot coals in his ear, the way he was so agitated. With the help of the nurse and his mom, we were able to get him onto the examining table and turn his head to one side so we could look down into his ear. There was blood on his fingers. The resident took his otoscope (the "ear thing" that we heard about at Cook County Hospital) and managed to look into his ear.

He turned to me and said, "This, you've got to see."

I took the otoscope and I made sure the light was working. I hovered over the little boy's ear. There was a giant bug in there! It had a dark brown shell and it was wiggling. As it moved, the boy screamed. I could see dried blood and fresh blood in the ear. The bug filled the entire ear canal. It was stuck.

I looked up at the resident and he said, "It's a roach. The Projects are full of them."

He motioned to the nurse and pointed to the bottle on a nearby counter.

It blew my mind. "Okay great, it's a roach. But how did it get in there?"

He put a couple of drops of an oily liquid in the boy's ear and then turned to me.

"When these kids sleep on the floor or on couches in those filthy apartments, the bugs crawl all over them at night, especially if they sleep on the floor. Sometimes the roaches fall into their external auditory canal and get stuck there."

I watched as he continued to drip the clear mineral oil down into the boy's ear. The roach stopped moving and the boy was settling down. After a couple of minutes, he took a pair of forceps and gently grasped the bug and pulled it out of the boy's ear. It was quite dead.

"Sometimes they really start digging in there and it when it scratches the eardrum, the kids go nuts with the pain."

As he stood there, I watched the nurse take the mom aside and show her the bottle of mineral oil that had been put in her little boy's ear. The emergency room couldn't cure poverty but they could teach the mothers how to help their children's suffering. Although it was a relatively minor injury, the sociological statement was enormous.

Lesson learned: It's bad to be poor.

ALMOST A FIASCO ON GRADUATION DAY

Up until that moment in my life, graduation from medical school was my very best day. Actually, it took two days. One day was the University graduation and the second day was the doctoral hooding ceremony for the medical school.

The diplomas were being given out by my recent Infectious Disease attending, Dr. George Gee Jackson. One of the things I learned on his service was that he had a great sense of humor.

I sat with my colleagues, awaiting the diploma and the handshake from Dr. Jackson. On my right ring finger was looped a trick windup buzzer from a practical joke store. My classmates were convinced that I would be thrown out of my own graduation, but I knew Dr. Jackson would get a kick out of it... I hoped.

My parents and family were sitting in the audience. My mother and father were bursting with pride. I could see my father getting out of his seat as he positioned himself at a strategic location at the side of the stage where I would be walking with my MD Diploma in hand. He had his Super-8 movie camera loaded and ready. He was going to fill that three-minute reel of film with my great moment.

Seeing my father's face was what made me unwind the buzzer and slip it back into my pocket. He was so proud of me; I couldn't let myself ruin it. Looking back, it was better that way. It was not the place for my stupid sense of humor.

The ceremonies passed like a blur and I was officially a Medical Doctor. In a few short years, I had gone from a lost graduate student with an uncertain future to being a doctor.

In medical school, I had gone from a green newbie to a guy about to become a Michael Reese Medical Intern in a couple of weeks. It was going to prove to be a hell of a year, as the next part of this book will show you.

PART III
INTERNSHIP AT MICHAEL REESE
MEDICAL CENTER, 1977

FINALLY, AN INTERN!

Medical school was finally finished and I was officially an MD... a doctor... or at least, an intern.

An intern (sometimes called a first-year medical resident), had a lot of responsibility at Michael Reese. We were supervised by a second-year resident, who in turn, was supervised by an attending who we met with each day.

Basically, the intern was the one who kept you alive while you were in the hospital. My fellow interns were the best of the best, carefully picked from many hundreds of applicants.

So far in this book, you have seen how medical school took me through all phases of medicine: surgery, ob/gyne, pediatrics, etcetera. At this next stage of training, things were now going to narrow down to medicine alone.

My time at Michael Reese would take me through all the subspecialties of medicine such as intensive care, cardiology, general medicine, emergency room, hematology, renal, and others. Although it may not seem obvious to some people, a good understanding in these disciplines is important for a neurologist, or for any other doctor for that matter. The nervous system is affected by every other part of the body.

A few days before the internship was to begin, I went to the Department of Medicine offices and got my schedule. Silly as it sounds, it seemed to make the internship seem more like a reality. Now I knew where it I would be each month. My first rotation was going to be the emergency room (ER). I was glad to see that, since I had finished my med school rotations in the same ER. I expected it would be an easy transition because I already knew the ropes.

From the Department of Medicine offices, I went to the Security office. They took my photograph and also took an impression of my fingerprints. I chuckled as I imagined that this was probably what it was like to get arrested and booked at the police station; at least that's the way they show it on television. (The photograph from that first ID badge appears on the cover of this book, along with the Michael Reese logo.) My last stop was to go down to the laundry through the tunnels to pick up my uniforms.

At one time, Michael Reese medical Center had 2400 beds, divided over many pavilions. Some of the pavilions were dedicated to research, but most were used for patient care. The entire complex, like many hospitals of the era, was connected by a complex underground tunnel system.

Those tunnels were a hotbed of activity. The tiled walls and the concrete floors echoed the hurried footsteps of doctors, nurses, technicians, and other employees. The air was filled with the rumble and squeals of rolling carts and large motorized industrial rolling flats. I already knew my way quite well through these busy tunnels, so I went directly down to the basement level and walked about 200 yards to where the laundry was located.

At that time, male interns at Michael Reese were required to wear white shirts and trousers, a short white jacket, and a tie. The female interns could choose between white slacks or white skirts. Of course, they didn't need to wear ties. At any time, we could drop our stuff off at the laundry and pick up a bundle of freshly pressed and starched uniforms.

Needless to say, we were constantly getting dirty with blood, Betadine, or strange unidentified body fluids. On call, we wore scrub suits, but by day we had to use our uniforms on regular patient rounds. I think the formality gave off a more professional impression... Besides, our Chairman insisted... Moreover, who were we to argue with Dr. Lou Sherwood?

Hokey as it sounds, it thrilled me to pick up my first bundle of uniforms. At that moment, I felt like I was officially a Michael Reese intern. You can laugh if you want.

THE EMERGENCY ROOM INTERN

In that era, before formal emergency room training was fully established, emergency rooms in the major teaching hospitals were staffed by people from medicine, surgery, and pediatrics. I personally think the care was excellent at that time, because the people truly knew what they were doing.

Because the Medicine department at Michael Reese dominated most of the medical center, and because our chairman, Dr. Louis Sherwood, believed in developing broad skills, the medicine intern was your first step if you came to the Michael Reese ER.

Surgeons would come down when summoned and pediatric patients were seen by pediatricians. Well before urgent care centers were conceived, Michael Reese had a fast track for minor emergencies such as sore throats and such. The fast track was manned by some older general practitioners hired for this purpose.

Any emergency more severe than a sore throat was seen by the Medicine house-staff. As one of the two new interns on the service, I was busy throughout my 12-hour shift. The ER was considered cushy because we actually got to go home for 12 hours when we were not working. This was not so on the inpatient services.

One of the eternal battles in a teaching hospital is the battle between the emergency room senior resident who wants to admit a patient to the floors and the on-call resident who is trying to keep his service from being overwhelmed.

During my first ER rotation, I had the opportunity to witness two very volatile personalities. Often their conversations would end with choice, witty repartees such as, "Fuck you, Marty." Followed by "No, fuck *you*, Harry."

I learned to take these battles in stride since I was not the one who had to fight with the admitting people. If I had a patient who needed to be admitted, assuming my resident agreed, he or she would take it from there. No one was sent home who needed to come in.

Peggy O was a classic ER nurse. She was a fixture in the emergency room. She was smart and delightfully sarcastic. I knew her from my student rotation in the ER, and I still have a lot of respect for her. She was smart and coolheaded, and she was the second most memorable nurse at Michael Reese. You will meet the first most memorable nurse later in this book.

THE ASSHOLE IN ROOM 7

I had just come on to the service, and I had not yet seen the first official patient of my internship. One of the older nurses walked up to me and said with a smug look, "Go see that asshole in Room 7." I just looked at her.

She laughed at my reaction. "Seriously, there's a guy with hemorrhoids in Room 7, and I want him out of here as soon as possible."

"Why the rush?" I was foolish enough to ask.

"Because that pimp son of a bitch came in by ambulance for his hemorrhoids! He took his Green Card out of his Crown Royal bag and took the damned ambulance! I'm getting sick of that shit."

The famed Green Card in those days was given by the welfare department to assure people proper medical care. They could go to any hospital they wanted. Unfortunately, it was greatly abused. The Crown Royal bag seemed to be a status symbol of some sort. I can see why the nurse was so angry. This sort of thing happened frequently. For some reason, people kept their Green Card in a Crown Royal bag.

I walked into Room 7, and indeed, the man looked like a Hollywood rendition of a pimp, right down to his fur-collared coat, which was thrown across a chair. He sat on the exam table and glared at me.

"About time," he said, looking at his gold watch. "I've got places to be and things to do," he complained to me.

Let's just say that he didn't make a very good first impression.

I asked him the appropriate questions, amidst his ongoing abusive dialog. I then examined him and told him the nurse would be back in a moment.

I walked out to the nursing desk, opened his chart, and *I WROTE MY FIRST PRESCRIPTION* that didn't need to be cosigned by a resident! As momentous as this occasion was, it was for the humble medication Anusol for the pimp's hemorrhoids. It's funny how you remember things like that. I'm sure the man was then able to move on, less painfully, to pursue his rewarding career as a purveyor of working girls. I don't know if he was able to get an ambulance to drive him back home again.

THE SLING AND THE KNIFE

My reverie didn't last long. Marty, my resident, sent me in to see a guy with a deep laceration. Apparently, he had been in a turf fight with a rival gang. Ortho already had fixed his dislocated left shoulder and immobilized it in a type of sling.

The Chicago Police Department had an unwritten policy that whenever they broke up gang fights, they wouldn't bring opposing gang members to the same hospital. For the most part, one gang would be sent to Michael Reese, and the other to Cook County Hospital. The nurses had told me that a couple of years earlier, there was an outright battle in the ER waiting room between two gangs. Apparently, it's a jungle out there.

I went into the room to see the guy with the laceration, and he was lying on the gurney with his left arm in a sling. He was scowling at me and didn't reciprocate when I gave him a cheerful hello. It might have been because his left ankle was cuffed to the rail of the gurney. He had a deep gash on his right upper leg that needed sutures. It was long and deep, but wasn't near any vital structures so I didn't need to call the surgeons in.

Standing next to him was a burly Chicago cop who looked extremely bored. "This guy got beaten up pretty good," he pointed to the leg. "Box cutter. You should see the other guy.... The ambulance took him over to County."

"So, why is he chained to the bed?"

"Well, this genius has a lot of outstanding warrants. I'm bringing him to lockup when you make him pretty again."

The nurses had already cut his pant leg off, given him a tetanus shot, set up the suture tray, and left the room. All I needed to do was stitch up that wound so the cops could bring him downtown. I opened the suture kit and snapped on my sterile gloves.

The patient continued to glare at me.

"I need to stitch up this leg, okay?"

He paused the proper "cool" duration of time and slowly nodded his approval of the plan. Very cool, indeed.

The bored cop looked at me and said, "Hey Doc, I gotta check something in my car. Okay? This guy's not going anywhere." I waved him out.

The patient said nothing, although he did wince when I injected the local anesthetic around his wound. I thoroughly cleaned the wound.

In addition to glaring at me, I could see him looking around the cubicle as I began placing absorbable stitches in the deeper parts of his wound. From the corner of my eye, I could see his right hand slowly moving into the sling on his left arm. He was pulling a knife out of the sling!

I didn't know what he was planning. Maybe a hostage situation. I didn't know and I didn't care.

I dropped my needle holder and grabbed his right arm with my sterile gloves, flipping it back. I had the mechanical advantage, and he couldn't use his left arm. His knife clattered to the floor. It looked like a Bowie knife as I remember it. It probably was a lot smaller, but my adrenaline was flowing at the time.

"A little help!" I yelled.

A nurse and an orderly rushed into the room, and a hospital security guard followed them in.

I had them hold him down while I put on some fresh gloves. He was struggling to get free and quietly issuing a stream of profanities. Before I resumed my stitching, I leaned over him and said into his ear, in my best John Wayne imitation, "You try that again and I'm gonna stitch your arm to this table."

I was shocked that he stopped struggling. One of the nurses snickered and I went back to my suturing job. I later felt somewhat guilty at what I had said to that felon. He had gotten the better of me.

Lesson learned: A doctor is not supposed to let emotions get in the way.

BROWN BAGGERS

The Michael Reese emergency room was a special place. By day, people of all walks of life would come through our doors. They ranged from the well-to-do executives working in the Chicago loop, to the downtrodden people who lived in the worsening neighborhoods around the hospital.

When there was a bus accident or a subway mishap in the area, hundreds of people would converge upon the emergency room. I always marveled that far more people would claim to be injured than you probably could fit on that bus or subway car which supposedly crashed or jumped a rail.

The waiting room was something to behold. On a quiet day, there usually were a couple of cops and dozens of people standing around, hands wrapped in bloody cloths or sitting in the waiting room chairs doubled over with abdominal pain and moaning. It was really no different from the Cook County emergency room. Children would be screaming and drunks would be swearing or puking into trashcans. It was the same drama.

The emergency room triage nurses were truly amazing. If you could see what they did in a single day, you would understand their cynicism.

No one is more cynical than a veteran emergency room nurse is. Like Peggy O, for example. She'd seen it all and she'd heard it all. She had a sixth sense about who needed to be seen immediately and who could wait. You couldn't bully her... I wouldn't even try.

One of the sad aspects of the Michael Reese emergency room, usually occurring at night was the appearance of a Brown Bagger.

The Brown Baggers would roll in on a gurney off an ambulance. Sometimes they would be mysteriously dropped off at the door of the emergency room by people who suddenly evaporated. The Brown Bagger was a sad testament to human cruelty and abandonment.

The Brown Bagger was usually an elderly person, usually demented, who was essentially left to the good will of the hospital. Their pathetic brown paper shopping bag would contain what was left of their earthly possessions, minus the valuables. These people were essentially being abandoned by their families. It was a one-way trip.

I dreaded the appearance of Brown Baggers, because deep inside, I knew that this was a person who was no longer loved. I also knew they would become a major placement problem, and we would have no clue about their past medical history. On rare occasion we would get lucky and they would tell us their full name so we could find a matching chart somewhere.

One Christmas Eve, I had three Brown Baggers to deal with. Merry Christmas. One was a man who just kept crying, and the other two were old women who had no idea where they were. The best we could do was to identify some kind of medical diagnosis and admit them to the proper service. The "proper service" usually ended up as 6 Main Reese. You'll hear more about this floor later.

THE MEAT WAGON

When dealing with the sociological problem of Brown Baggers, it was sometimes a welcome change, sadly, when the cops pulled around the back of the ER with their Meat Wagon. This was a white Chicago PD paddy wagon with one or more corpses in it, needing to be officially pronounced dead.

The irony was that I would be looking at someone frozen solid or in rigor mortis, and the official time of death would be the moment when I pronounced them. Some of these deliveries were more interesting than others.

One time, for example, they paged me out to the Meat Wagon to pronounce a man who had just been shot. Cops are cynical, like ER nurses, and they have a dark sense of humor. They are like medical people... we essentially see the same awful things. They just see them first.

I walked out the back door of the ER and I noted that they had backed up the Meat Wagon to our door.

Cop #1 slammed the driver's door and walked back to me, smiling.

"Hi Doc. It looks like we're back again with another good one for you."

Cop #2 came around the other side of the truck. "Yeah. This one's a piece of work. He's got a rap sheet longer than your arm."

Cop #1 gripped the handle on the rear door of the paddy wagon, saying, "He broke into an old lady's apartment a couple of weeks ago. Actually, we took the call, right Charlie?"

"You got that right, buddy. This son-of-a-bitch beat the crap out of an old lady. He pulled her out of her wheelchair and then he raped her. That was two weeks ago."

They were trying for the classic dramatic buildup, but I was starting to get cold. I walked to the back door of the Meat Wagon and asked them what they wanted to hear. "So, why is he here now?"

The cops both chuckled, enjoying the suspense. I was freezing, and I wanted to get to the end of the story.

Cop #1 took over. "Today, he broke down her door again. Again! This time when he went charging into the room...," he paused for effect, "... she pulled out a .38 snub nose from her wheelchair and popped him square in the forehead."

At this point in the story, the cops, with their dark sense of drama, unlatched the back of the paddy wagon and swung open the doors. The dead man had a .38 caliber hole dead center in his forehead, like a Hindu bindi dot. He also had a very surprised expression on his face. This image remains burned in my memory. Maybe there is justice after all.

Cop #2 laughed. "Now, tell me Doc, is that one surprised lookin' son-of-a-bitch or what?"

They both laughed. I must say, I enjoyed the irony.

Other Meat Wagon deliveries were somewhat dubious. On another brisk winter day, I was shivering in my short-sleeved scrub suit as I followed the cops out to the wagon. They had brought me a man with several holes drilled on each side of his head.... probably from a 1/4" power drill. There was a great deal of dried blood on his scalp and face.

"Another suicide, Doc," the first officer told me. "We found him with the Black & Decker drill still in his hand."

"How can you call that a suicide? Even the first hole would probably have killed him. There's no way that's a suicide."

The cop was quite adamant. "No. That's a suicide."

I signed his paperwork and they took off with the perforated man. It was my theory that they didn't want to investigate it.

Lesson learned: If you decide to kill yourself, leave a note.

THE LADY WITH THE CATS

For the sake of privacy, we will call this lady Cassie Wilson. Mrs. Wilson was an elderly black woman who was widowed for many years. She lived in the projects on the South Side of Chicago, and had taken a bus to the hospital because she was having trouble breathing. She must have looked pretty bad when she huffed into the ER reception area, because the triage nurses grabbed her, loaded her onto a gurney, and quickly pushed her into one of the ER bays.

When I saw her rolling in, I went right over to her. The nurses had already propped up the back of the gurney to an almost sitting position so she could breathe more comfortably. She could only talk in short phrases because she was badly short of breath. I ordered some labs and drew blood gases from her radial artery while telling a student nurse to put her on nasal prongs with 4 liters of oxygen. Soon, she was a little more comfortable and able to talk in more detail. We pulled the curtains around the gurney and hooked her up to a cardiac monitor.

When she was more comfortable and the labs were cooking, we began to talk.

She said that for the last few days she had been having chest pain and shortness of breath. She pointed down to her feet, which were swollen well above her ankles.

"I'm embarrassed, Doctor."

"Why is that?"

"Well, I can't wear my good shoes no more. My feet are too swollen. I had to wear my house slippers to come here."

"You don't need to apologize for that. Slippers are fine."

She was a sweet old lady and appeared very worried about something else. She didn't say what.

"Mrs. Wilson," I asked, "do you have any family in the area?"

"No, I don't have any family around here... Just my people from church. They're like my family."

"No kids at all?"

"I've got one son living... But he's in jail."

I didn't ask why. I listened to her heart and lungs. She was obviously in congestive heart failure.

Soon, she was breathing better on the oxygen and the diuretic I gave her, but she was still short of breath. She started talking again.

"I live in the projects. You know the projects?"

"Yes, I do. I drive past them when I come up the Dan Ryan."

"I live on the fifth floor."

The nurse was attaching electrocardiogram leads to her chest as we were talking. I was looking at the tracing as Mrs. Wilson continued to talk.

"I don't take the elevator. Those boys rob people in the elevators."

I knew what she meant; there was a great deal of crime in the projects. Mostly young toughs and druggies.

"So, how do you get up to your apartment?"

"Usually, I take the stairs. It takes a long time but I don't want nobody mugging me."

Five flights was quite a distance to climb, especially for a woman of her age. I steered the conversation to a medically relevant point.

"How well do you handle five flights of stairs?"

She laughed. "Not so good. I been getting short of breath. Have to stop at each landing for a while to catch my breath."

"Does it make your chest hurt when you climb the stairs?"

"Sometimes. Especially yesterday. I didn't think I would make it.... But I did. I had to... a lot of pressure."

My supervising resident, Sarcastic Stu, stuck his head through the curtain and solemnly motioned me out. I excused myself and led him out of earshot. I presented Cassie Wilson's case to him.

"Okay," he said in his usual curt way, "so she's in failure?"

I nodded. "Yeah, but no acute changes on EKG."

"So, admit her to 6 East and let's get moving. They're starting to pile up out there. What did you do so far?"

"I got her on O2, started an IV and pushed 40 of Lasix."

"Okay, so, again, admit her. Chop chop."

He rushed away to call the admitting service on call. The plan was to put Cassie on the medical floor to stabilize her and find out why she was in failure. It was my job to go back and tell her the news.

Cassie flatly refused to be admitted. She wouldn't tell me why. She seemed very disappointed in me and struggled to swing her swollen legs over the edge of the table. Her mottled legs and swollen feet dangled over the edge with her sad, worn-out slippers almost falling off.

I tried to reason with her. "Mrs. Wilson, you're very sick and you need to be in the hospital." She crossed her arms and turned her head away from me.

"You're in heart failure!"

She shook her head and I noticed that her wig was not quite on straight.

I almost pleaded with her. "Mrs. Wilson, seriously, this is not going to cost you anything. It's a public hospital!"

She turned toward me, saying, "There is just no way I'm coming into this hospital."

"Why not? You're sick. Look how hard it is for you to breathe."

She raised her voice. "I just can't! Just give me some medicines and send me on my way. What's wrong with you, Doctor?"

She was winded after that tirade. She was trying to catch her breath when Sarcastic Stu came up to me, talking as if the Cassie wasn't even there.

"Messina, what's the holdup? Why is she still here?"

I motioned him away from the gurney but he stopped me after about 10 feet.

"Messina, don't tell me that you can't convince this little old lady to come into the hospital for a couple of nights. Is that what you're trying to tell me?"

"Stu, she just won't come in no matter what I say."

As we talked, looking over Stu's shoulder, I could see Cassie pulling off her oxygen prongs. She was clearly ready to leave. She was looking around for her clothing and then started fumbling behind her neck to untie her hospital gown.

Stu looked at me as if I was an idiot. "Come here and watch this."

He was going to be a big shot and show this stupid intern a few things. He walked over to Mrs. Cassie Wilson.

"What's the problem here... er Cassie?" He said condescendingly, "Don't you like our hospital?"

For such a sweet old lady, she gave Stu one hell of a dirty look which stopped him in his tracks. Then, she waved him away. Stu walked away scowling, impatiently motioning me toward her again to try to talk some sense into her.

I went back to her bedside and smiled at her. She was struggling to breathe again. I gently placed her oxygen prongs in her nostrils and looped the green tubing over her ears. She didn't fight me. I started with some small talk and soon, we were chatting.

She was softening up, asking me, "Are you a full-fledged doctor?"

"No, ma'am, I'm an intern."

"I had a lot of hopes for my son, Lavern. I don't know where I went wrong."

I didn't say anything.

"You know, all I have in the world are my two cats." She laughed. "Their names are Billy-Bob and Bobby-Bob."

I laughed with her. I knew what kind of statement she was making, in her own way. She had grown up in rural Mississippi and was getting even.

"Billy-Bob is a red cat and Bobby-Bob is what they call a tuxedo cat. I have a picture somewheres." She looked around to see where her things were.

"You really love those cats, don't you?"

She turned back to me. "I sure do. Sometimes they play and sometimes they fight. But I know they love each other. Just like I love them both."

"They stay in your apartment with you?"

"They sure do! I'd never let them out. Sometimes, when I can," She laughed, "I use my food stamps to buy them tuna. They come running when they hear that can opener turnin'."

Peggy, the ER charge nurse, was giving me dirty looks and pointing upward, frowning, and mouthing the words "Admit her."

I just waved to her and daggers flashed from her eyes. I shrugged and she made a gesture as if she was slitting her throat. Then she pointed at me.

After I was properly blasted, Peggy moved on to the next bed and I turned back to Mrs. Cassie Wilson.

Cassie could sense that I was being pressured and she motioned me to come closer. She was trying to say something but I couldn't hear her because of the ER noise and chaos all around us. I came closer.

"I can't come into the hospital because of my cats."

"I don't understand."

"I said I can't come in because of my cats."

I shouted over the noise of a drunk yelling in the next bed. "No, what I mean is, why *can't* you come in?"

"I've got a neighbor, Mr. Davis. He's a pretty bad man and he's gonna rob my apartment if he finds out I'm in the hospital. I just know it. He's gonna break down my door and then my cats'll run away."

It dawned on me, finally. She was willing to risk her health for the sake of Billy-Bob and Bobby-Bob.

I patted her on the arm and smiled, saying, "Don't go anywhere. I'll be right back."

She settled back and watched me walk away. She left the oxygen prongs in place and waited.

When I was out of sight of Cassie, I took a deep breath and sadly realized how awful this woman's life was.

Stu came up to me and said, "What are you waiting for? Either she signs out against advice or she gets admitted. Which will it be?"

"I'm working on it, give me a few minutes."

Just then, Stu was paged and he swore and stormed away. From the corner of my eye, I could see Mary-The-Social-Worker.

Through a combination of luck and what I'd like to think was charm, I convinced Mary to find a cat watcher. She talked to Cassie and got the number of her pastor.

Despite the escalating wrath of Peggy and Stu, I held firm until Mary gave her the good news. Cassie then agreed to be admitted to the floor known as "6 East, Main Reese." She waved to me and smiled as her gurney rolled past the desk to the elevator.

That was the last time I saw Cassie Wilson. She died the next day. I remember hoping that her church family would look after Billy-Bob and Bobby-Bob.

MAGGOTS

When things were quiet in the ER, on rare occasion, we would send for pizza from Connie's Pizza on Cottage Grove, which was right near the hospital.

On such a night, I was wolfing down a pizza with the nurses and other house-staff when someone brought up the topic of "What's the most disgusting thing you've ever smelled?"

I had played that game before; apparently, it's a common pastime among the cynical ER crowd. The contenders included smelly rednecks, incontinent winos, an autopsy on a "floater" (drowning victim), and others. Pretty much everyone agreed that a dead leg had probably the most disgusting odor. This referred to a gangrenous limb, which was caused by peripheral arterial disease or infections in uncontrolled diabetics or heavy smokers.

The conversation made its way over to the grossest things we've ever seen and decubitus ulcers came up.

A decubitus ulcer is a deep bedsore that is found on the sacrum or buttocks of a person who has been essentially abandoned. Such people are left to lie in bed and not be washed or turned. The decubitus ulcers look like craters.

Stu piped up, "You know, the topping on this pizza looks very much like a deep decubitus ulcer, except for the green pus. Maybe we should have ordered some guacamole topping."

None of us were particularly disgusted or grossed out, and Stu looked disappointed.

A few days after this deep intellectual discussion, an obese woman was brought in from a local nursing home, supposedly because her diabetes was out of control. She was severely demented and lethargic, slowly looking around the room and at me as I walked up to her.

I smiled a greeting and pulled back her blanket to examine her. I was literally stopped in my tracks by the intense odor of rotting flesh, and I had been around some nasty things in my life. Her left foot was almost black with gangrene. As I was looking at the leg, I thought I saw something move. I didn't really believe it, so I stared a bit longer. Surely enough, I could see movement on the irregular surface of that black foot.

Flies lay eggs that become maggots, and maggots grow up to become flies. The woman had maggots in her foot. Apparently, flies had laid eggs in the dying flesh, and they had hatched into maggots. I had heard stories of maggots cleaning wounds such as decubitus ulcers, but these creatures were just living in her dead foot, eating the dead flesh. The smell was awful.

I completed my evaluation, drew some blood, and brought my resident over to see her. My resident then brought the medicine attending over. As I recall, the nurses kept some potassium permanganate in the ER, and they painted the purple liquid on her dead foot. Apparently, various types of worms and larvae do not like this chemical. Indeed, some of the maggots came to the surface.

Incidentally, have you ever wondered how a fly can be buzzing around you in your favorite restaurant in the dead of winter? Certainly, it didn't fly in from outdoors. Remember, today's fly was yesterday's maggot. It might be best not to look in the restaurant's kitchen.

Lessons learned: Do not be surprised when people neglect people. Don't eat in restaurants plagued by flies in the wintertime.

IN THE NICK OF TIME

On the last night of my ER rotation, all hell was breaking loose, both on the Southside of Chicago and in the Michael Reese Emergency Room. There were gunshot wounds and knife wounds galore, and in the middle of this, the Chicago Fire Department pulled up with their big, square, red rescue truck. These were like super ambulances, and the paramedics were top-notch. Even after all these years, I've never seen better.

They were pushing a stretcher through the sliding door, and on it lay a woman who appeared to be in her late 40s. One of the paramedics was doing chest compressions, and the other was holding a mask against her face and squeezing an Ambu bag to breathe for her (paramedics didn't intubate in those days). We moved into action fast. As two nurses and I were pulling her from the stretcher onto the emergency room table, the paramedic who was compressing her chest breathlessly told us her story.

"This lady was just walking down the street near Goldblatt's when she just collapsed on the sidewalk. A cop was standing there and saw her go down, so he called it in."

I took over the compressions to give the guy a break while he talked.

"We were just around the corner when the call came in. Lucky break.

"She wasn't down for very long because we started working on her right away. We immediately started resuscitation. Here, Doc, let me take over again."

With all the madness around us, it turned out that I was the only doctor available... Everyone else was seriously tied up with other crises. By now, I had been on many codes for cardiac arrests.

I immediately started giving orders for an IV and cardiac monitor. The ER nurses, of course, knew exactly what I was going to ask for and everything was happening fast and competently.

I stood at the head of the table and stretched the woman's head back. I slipped the laryngoscope down the back of her throat. The endotracheal tube slid easily down her trachea and one of the nurses immediately inflated the cuff, which makes a tight seal in the airway. The other nurse was taping the tube to her face so it wouldn't slip out. A respiratory therapist was now squeezing the Ambu bag.

Chicago's Bravest were continuing their chest compressions until I took over again. Looking quickly around the room, I was still the only house officer available. I looked at the cardiac monitor and could see no useful rhythm. I ordered more meds to be pushed into the IV, stopped, and zapped her with the defibrillator. We then continued the standard procedure ...compressing her chest, pushing meds, and breathing for her.

It seemed like we were working on her for a long time, but I was absolutely committed and would not give up. She looked too young to be having a heart attack, and I would be damned if I was going to lose this patient. I continued pushing drugs, zapping her with the defibrillator, and continued the frantic and dramatic procedure. The nurses were looking at each other with "that look," and I felt very self-conscious at being the newbie who didn't know when to quit. But... I was *not* going to quit.

It seemed almost like magic when her heart flipped into a normal sinus rhythm, and pretty soon we could actually palpate a pulse in her neck. I got big smiles from the nurses as they taped her IVs into position and covered her chest in the name of modesty (as if modesty really existed in an emergency room... Let's call it dignity).

The ER was quieting down. I could hear less hubbub from the other treatment bays. My senior resident finally came over, gave me a pat on the back, and kept going to the next bay. I sat at this lady's bedside, looking at her and her monitor as the nurses went through her purse and finally got a name.

For the sake of her privacy, let's call her Carol. She lived in the projects on the south side of Chicago. These buildings were subsidized housing units, and violent crime was rampant, due in part to the drug trade. Carol lived in one of these places.

Other than the fact that we were able to save Carol's life, another big miracle for that day was the fact that her purse was still with her as she lay helpless on the sidewalk... Moreover, it actually contained her wallet. She was one lucky lady. Except, of course, for the heart attack.

I continued to sit and proudly watch Carol's heartbeat on the heart monitor as my adrenaline surge began to come down. My feelings of desperate excitement were receding and I was feeling pretty darned good about myself.

My reverie was broken when the ER charge nurse came over to me.

"They've got a bed in the CCU (Cardiac Care Unit) and we're getting ready to transfer her."

She smiled. Earning respect from the experienced ER nurses is one of the hardest things in medicine.

Then she said, "Now it's time to get off your ass because we're getting backed up out there."

Nevertheless, it was a good feeling.

The rest of the shift went on like a usual Friday night on the Southside; it was never dull. I had my share of lacerations, bladder infections, and a few people with nasty venereal diseases. It was turning into a typical Friday night, and it was my last night on this service. I almost hated to leave; they were a good crew to work with.

THE WOMAN WHO REMEMBERED ME

The following day, I started my CCU rotation. The CCU at Michael Reese was an amazing place. We had the latest equipment from Hewlett-Packard. In fact, our cardiac management system was a prototype at the time. It was the only one in the country. There were about 14 beds as I recall, which were connected to this master system. They were all full.

I had almost no sleep the night before, and here I was at 7:00 AM taking report from my fellow intern, Steve, who was now coming off the service. He looked like hell. We all looked like hell that year.

"Well, Ed," he said, while sucking down some black coffee in the conference room, "I can't say that I'm sad to leave this service." He grinned, "Today I start my endocrinology elective and there's no call."

The senior resident on the service, Mary, walked into the room and looked at the two of us standing there.

"Hi boys. Well, shall we start?"

The three of us walked from bed to bed as Steve told me about each person, Mary nodding agreement as he spoke. Steve was a damned good doctor and I felt lucky to inherit his patients. They were always well worked up and tuned. Mary was a good senior resident, and I was glad to be able to work with her. Steve later became a world famous cardiologist.

We got to Room 5, and I recognized Carol's name on the door.

Steve got a big smile on his face. "Carol here is a 51-year-old black female who had a large inferior wall MI [myocardial infarction, heart attack]. She's got a great rhythm and blood pressure, and barely has needed any pressor agents. She's pretty much breathing on her own, so you could probably extubate her pretty soon. A true success story."

I looked in the room and there was Carol attached to the Bennett MA-1 ventilator. Above her head, the cardiac monitor showed a beautiful, normal rhythm and pressures.

We continued our journey from room to room, and I scribbled detailed notes from what Steve was saying. There were many unstable people on the service and Steve warned me about the attending cardiologist who was a ball breaker. I'll call him Dr. G for the sake of his privacy.

"Dr. G will be here before you know it, so you'd better review these charts." Steve smirked and Mary looked away.

I spent the rest of the day memorizing everyone's chart and putting out fires with Mary's help for people with congestive heart failure, unstable angina, and dangerous heart rhythms. Mary transferred one of our most stable patients out to the intermediate care unit, and we admitted a new person from the ER.

Things were tough and we didn't get much sleep that night. Carol was doing pretty well. We had her off the ventilator but we kept her endotracheal tube in place for the night. I could tell she didn't like it, but it was bad luck to extubate people late in the day.

The next morning after work rounds, Mary and I pulled out Carol's endotracheal tube, and after the usual coughing and swearing, we could see that Carol was quite stable. She smiled at us as Mary and I left the room and moved on to our next challenge, leaving her to the nurses and the respiratory therapist.

We finished work rounds and had our usual encounter with Dr. G, the cardiology attending, who seemed to have an unlimited supply of trick questions to ask me about each patient. I honestly think he was trying to be a good teacher, using the time-honored teaching method known as "teaching by intimidation."

A few hours later, I went back to check on Carol. The nurse had cranked up the head of the bed and she had a tray in front of her. She was grinning at me.

"Hey Doc. When do I get real food?" She pointed to the clear liquid diet on her tray.

I sat down on the chair next to her bed. "Sorry about the clear liquids, we just had to make sure you weren't going to choke. I think when you begin to complain about the food, it's time to advance your diet."

I had her chart on my lap and I wrote an order for her to advance to a solid cardiac diet. I closed the chart and I stood up next to her bed.

"Carol, please excuse my manners. I never actually introduced myself. I'm Dr. Messina, and I'll be the intern taking care of you in the heart unit."

"I know who you are," she said looking directly into my eyes, "you're the guy from the emergency room."

I just looked at her. I didn't know how she knew that. In those days, the Michael Reese interns pretty much all looked alike and dressed alike, except for the female interns.

"What do you mean, Carol?"

"I mean, you're the guy who was pounding so hard on my chest and shocking me with that machine." She rubbed her sternum and made a painful face.

I sat back down again. "How could you know that? You were unconscious the whole time."

"Well, it was you, right?" She asked, and I nodded.

"I knew it! Well, it's kind of funny. I felt like I was floating above everything. It was like I was on the ceiling, looking down. I could see myself lying there and you and the others were all over me."

She stopped and reached out to touch my hand, earnestly saying, "I'm glad you didn't give up."

About halfway through this conversation, one of the CCU nurses, Kathy, had come into the room to pass meds and she stopped when she heard what Carol was saying. I motioned her in while Carol continued.

"It was the craziest thing," she continued. "At the same time, I was floating on a boat, down a river made of light. There were tall cliffs on either side with bright a big light at the end of the river. There were people up high on the cliffs and I know they were far away, but I knew who they were."

She paused and got tearful.

"I could see my grandmother and my Daddy."

She turned toward the nurse, explaining "They both died when I was little."

She turned back to me and continued, "They kept yellin' to me... They kept saying 'turn back...turn back'... It was the craziest thing. Then, I don't remember a single thing until I woke up in here with that tube in my throat." she said, motioning around the room.

We spoke a bit more and then the nurse and I left the room.

When we got back out to the desk, Kathy and I both sat down with the charts; we didn't know what to say to each other.

To this day, I believe Carol was telling us the truth, and I still puzzle about how was she able to recognize me from when she was unconscious. I will leave this for others to evaluate... perhaps those who have read Elisabeth Kubler-Ross's book, On Death and Dying. When I asked her later that day, Carol didn't know who that was.

Lesson learned: there's hope.

THE MAN WITH THE ANKLE

Not every day was dramatic on the CCU. Nor was it always easy to get information from a patient. One day, the ER admitted an elderly Polish gentleman whose larynx had been removed the previous year because of throat cancer. His only way of speaking was with a vibrating speech device, which he held to his throat. Unfortunately when he had his heart attack, the paramedics didn't bring that device with him. His family was supposed to bring it the next day, but it was midnight and I needed to take a history.

A good deal of the questions I could ask had a yes or no answer, so we got along pretty well. When I asked him what else was bothering him he pointed to his left ankle. When I did my examination, I paid particular attention to his ankle. It was not painful or swollen, and the foot was not paralyzed, discolored, or deformed. I kept asking him, "What do you mean?" He tried to mouth some words that I could not understand. He kept pointing down to his ankle, getting very frustrated.

It dawned on me that he could probably write it down for me. It turned out that he was illiterate. He had come from a small village in Poland before the War, and had never learned to read and write. What were the odds?

I had the nurse come in and try to find out what he meant. She walked out of the room, shaking her head from side to side. I even asked my senior resident to go in and try to find out what he meant by pointing to his left ankle. Nothing.

I was going to let it go until the morning when his family was going to come in with his speaking device. In the meantime, he was stable so I didn't sweat it. I kept thinking about what he was trying to tell me about his left ankle.

The following day was busy; I made rounds on this gentleman first thing in the morning, and didn't get back to him until about noon since he was so stable. We were going to transfer him to the step-down unit in another day.

Finally, I got back to his room and he was smiling, holding up his talking device. Kathy and I walked over to his bed.

"So, I see your family brought in the buzzer."

With the artificial, almost robotic sound, he said, with his accent, "Yes. Finally, I make people to understand me."

"So now, can you please tell me why you were pointing to your left ankle? This has been driving me crazy, you know. What the heck were you trying to tell me?"

He looked at me, pointing again to his left ankle and said, with his buzzing voice, "I have trouble to control bladder. Piss keeps going down left leg." He looked at me with frustration, "Now, you help me?"

Kathy and I looked at each other, and it was almost impossible to suppress a laugh. Certainly, it was not to make fun of this poor man, but the fact that we didn't understand his pantomime.

Lesson learned: Communication is important, and some people aren't very good at it.

FALLING ASLEEP IN THE CONFERENCE

Throughout the following day, we were discharging and transferring patients out of the CCU like mad. We were naturally glad when people get better, but then we would then be swamped with new admissions from the ER until our empty beds were full again.

That's exactly what happened that night. Mary, my resident, and I were up all night long without a wink of sleep. Night call in the CCU meant that you literally slept in the unit's call room. You did not leave the CCU for any reason, and you ordered a food tray from the dietary service, as if you were a patient.

You could order anything you wanted except the lobster, unless it was a holiday. Yes, lobster. Food Service had some good food because of the private patients, and the doctors ate well on CCU and ICU call. The irony was that we barely got to touch our food that evening; the trays got cold and we tried to salvage the least disgusting parts, chewing as we feverishly wrote our notes.

If there had been a choice between eating a meal and getting fifteen minutes of sleep, I would have chosen the sleep. By the time we got everybody worked up and stabilized, I was completely exhausted. Mary and I went into the small kitchen to suck down some black coffee so we could survive the next eight hours when Dr. G, the attending cardiologist, burst into the room.

"Messina, did you prepare the cases you're going to present at the arrhythmia conference?" He held up his watch..."It's in ten minutes."

Mary looked at me as if my dog had died. She was feeling my pain...

Dr. G pressed on, "You'd *better* do me proud. Our guests are legends... They practically invented the EKG! Have you at least read their book on cardiac arrhythmias?"

The book to which he was referring was about three inches thick, and apparently it was like a Bible to cardiologists. There was no time when I could possibly have read it, and frankly, it wasn't exactly on my list of leisure reading as a future neurologist.

Mercifully for Mary, she had to run down to the ER for a new admission with unstable angina. I was on my own. I didn't have any time to prepare these patient presentations because Dr. G had just told me about it about 24 hours earlier. There had been no time.

The conference room, if you could call it that, was about 12 x 12 with a large table in the middle surrounded by chairs. I was to sit at the far end, possibly to prevent my escape. Dr. G ushered in the two world-renowned arrhythmia experts to sit across from each other, and Dr. G sat on my right to see that the cases were "handled properly." These pleasant elderly European men were medical legends who had done much of their work at Michael Reese in years past.

I knew that my brain needed sleep or it would not function. I had already downed one cup of black coffee when Dr. G had burst onto the scene, and I carried another one into the conference room. Dr. G saw the cup and told me, "Lose the coffee... sign of disrespect."

Before I could even reach to dump the black liquid down my esophagus, he grabbed the cup and dropped it into a nearby receptacle. I was screwed.

After the distinguished professors were seated, some of the other cardio attendings joined us. The room was packed, and it was hot and stuffy. No windows.

The plan was for me to read the case summaries from these patients' previous admissions and demonstrate the abnormal cardiac rhythms from the cardiograph strips that were pasted in the charts. I groaned when I saw the stack of charts. (Paper strips and paper charts were the norm in those days.)

The distinguished professors were to take the paper rhythm strips and comment on each one, showing how they would have interpreted them. These brilliant men spoke slowly and methodically with very thick accents... in a low monotone. They were known for their fastidious ways, and each produced a small EKG ruler from their pocket. They methodically measured the blips on those tracings as I passed them over to them.

They would look each other if a wave, duration, or complex was out of the ordinary. If someone asked a question, the professors would go into great detail, taking turns explaining their answers.

I imagine that this would have been wonderful, probably a world class experience, had I been a cardiology fellow. Unfortunately, I was unable to resist the heat, the monotonous vocal tones, and the lack of relevance... I began to nod off as I was trying very hard to be polite and attentive. If my head nodded down, I would experience a severe pain in my right rib cage as Dr. G fiercely elbowed me, his fiery glance shooting daggers into my drooping eyes. These were his mentors.

The ordeal repeated itself; reading, nodding, rib pain. This cycle went on for at least an hour. Eventually, it was over! Everyone began filing out of the tiny, overheated room. The cool air outside the conference room was wonderful.

As Dr. G walked out with the two professors, he was briefly pulled aside by Mary who needed to tell him about a patient in the ER. She was saving me from his wrath, bless her heart.

I managed to catch up with our esteemed guests and apologized for my sleepiness, explaining about the night before. They were quite gracious and told me they certainly understood. I felt much better because it's important to respect those who deserve it. Unfortunately, Dr. G was on my case for the duration of my rotation. I knew he couldn't hurt me because I already was locked into my Washington University neurology residency, but it still was uncomfortable.

Dr. G was known as a great cardiologist and an excellent teacher, as I later discovered. I felt bad that we had gotten off on the wrong foot.

Lesson learned: Sometimes circumstances take over and there is nothing you can do about it.

THE MOUSE

The CCU wasn't all fun and games, but it had its light moments. It seems that when you are chronically sleep deprived and under massive amounts of life-and-death stress, non-funny things might strike you funny.

The Michael Reese CCU was a modern wonder of its time. The many glass-fronted individual rooms were located in a large oval. Long nursing desks and rows of monitoring equipment ran down the middle. It was almost a brand new unit. The building which contained the new CCU was considerably older, which explains the rest of my story.

The second-year resident rotations changed on this particular day. My new resident was Paul Bernstein. He told me that the new patient being admitted seemed anxious, and suggested that it might be better if the two of us went in together to take her history and do our examinations.

We both went into the room, and Paul pulled out a chair near the foot of her bed. I sat next to the bed. The beds in the CCU were cranked up higher than usual hospital beds for reasons I never understood. At any rate, the patient was an elderly, nervous woman who was scared to death because she had just had a heart attack.

She was new to the hospital, so we didn't have previous records, meaning that the detailed general history was going to take longer than it would for an established patient. As Paul started the questioning, I began jotting notes, occasionally interjecting a question for clarification. As I looked down to the chart on my lap, I noted that a little brown mouse was running across the room. Because the patient was up so high, she didn't see it from where she was.

As our nervous patient was talking, the last thing I needed to do was to give her another heart attack. I tried to be subtle, waving to Paul and pointing down at the floor. He didn't seem to get it and continued asking her questions. I coughed to get his attention and pointed down again. He glanced down just as the mouse was zooming out from under the bed. The poor little furry dude was clearly lost.

Finally, Paul caught on and he nonchalantly took an empty Styrofoam cup from the patient's tray table, as if he were just looking at it, turning it over in his hand. I continued the questioning, diverting her attention from Paul as he held the cup upside down and leaned to one side so he could perhaps trap the mouse against the floor if it scooted past him.

Like I said, I was getting somewhat punchy from sleep deprivation, and I was trying very hard not to laugh. This was particularly difficult because the patient was telling me in all sincerity about her symptoms, with me trying to lock her gaze so she wouldn't see Paul trying to catch that mouse.

Thankfully, the mouse found the open door and fled the patient's room. Apparently, the nurses didn't notice the little fellow, and he probably found his way home. I'm certain that this was not a hallucination because Paul and I went to the break room and couldn't stop laughing about it.

Lesson learned: Control your facial expressions; you never know when a mouse will run by.

THE MEDICAL ICU

When my stint in the CCU was finished, my next rotation was the general medical ICU (intensive care unit). That made two intense rotations back to back. Unfortunately, the resident who was going to be assigned to me had been in a serious car accident and had to be hospitalized. He had been driving home after being on call, totally exhausted, and he fell asleep and hit a tree on Lakeshore Drive. He broke a lot of bones but could have been killed.

For this reason, the usual team of one intern and one resident had to be altered. The resident covering a nearby medical floor was also going to available to me as needed. Like the CCU rotation, I had to sleep on the unit and my meal trays were brought to me by dietary.

Teaching was constant in the ICU. There were frequent teaching rounds from the director of the ICU, the anesthesiologists who checked on the ventilators, the medicine attendings, and the surgical attendings. In addition, there were numerous consult teams coming through such as Renal, Cardiology, Infectious Disease, Pulmonary and Anesthesiology. Everyone had something to teach and I loved it. What I learned in my two rotations in the ICU came in very handy in later years.

The ICU should have been called the ITU, for "Intensive Teaching Unit."

Like the other floors at Michael Reese, the ICU had a great nursing staff and the most organized unit clerk I had ever seen. She was a take-charge person, and nothing got past her. I'm embarrassed that I don't remember her name, so I'll call her Miss Pettigrew. I do remember that she insisted on being called "Miss" plus her last name. She was very professional.

As proof that we live in a small world, one of the ICU nurses was Mary O, sister of the famed ER nurse, Peggy O. What were the odds that one family would produce two great nurses?

The Michael Reese ICU was a large open area with ten medical and ten surgical ICU beds. The nurses were cross-trained and felt comfortable on either side. Unfortunately, they didn't have much confidence in the surgical intern who was covering the surgical beds.

I was grateful that in my fourth year of medical school, I had been a sub-intern in General Surgery at the University of Illinois Hospital under Dr. Robert Baker. He was the master of fluids and electrolytes, and his teaching came in very handy.

The surgical attendings preferred to have the Medicine service co-manage their ICU patients, so basically, when I was on duty, I was looking after about 20 beds instead of eight.

I had a 12-hour break from the time I left the CCU until I began my ICU rotation and I felt more exposed because I did not have an on-site resident to work with me.

TETANUS

On my second day, the surgeons sent us a man with tetanus. He was a 30-year-old Haitian who had never been vaccinated. He was living on the South Side and was helping someone clear an empty lot when he cut his leg on something nasty. He didn't consider it a major cut, so he didn't seek medical attention at the time.

A few days later, his friends brought him into the ER because of abdominal spasms, and he offhandedly mentioned that his leg was becoming infected. The ER resident called the surgical service who admitted him to the general surgery floor to observe him for the abdominal pain and to debride (cutting away dead tissue) and treat his leg infection. The following day, the nurses observed that he had trouble opening his jaw, and he was drooling.

Neurology evaluated him and transferred him to the ICU. They preferred that he be on the medical side of the unit with the surgeons consulting on wound management. By now, the surgeons had decided to extend the debridement of the wound. He was started on tetanus immune globulin.

The man's muscle spasms progressed rapidly, and soon he was tensing up his back muscles so much that he was painfully bending backward. I started him on a Valium IV drip.

He kept worsening. Even the slightest sound or touch would send him into painful spasms. I was worried that if I kept pushing up the Valium, he would stop breathing. On the other hand, we were afraid that he would begin tearing muscles and fracturing bones.

We intubated him and placed him on a ventilator. This way, we could assure breathing while we used strong muscle relaxing, respiratory suppressing medications. We kept him in a dark room, and the nurses would push extra doses of Valium when they were handling him. He was sensitive to any type of stimulus. The idea was to keep him from hurting himself until the crisis was over.

I noticed on a portable chest x-ray that he had a fresh compression fracture of one of his vertebrae, probably from one of those powerful muscle spasms.

I recall reading somewhere that sometime after the Civil War, the designer of the Brooklyn Bridge, John Roebling, died of tetanus. He had sustained a crush injury to his foot when surveying the location of the great bridge. He would not let the doctors treat him and he died a terrible and painful death.

Lesson learned: Tetanus is nothing to be trifled with. Get your shots!

THE DREAM

One night, while I was attempting sleep in the ICU call room, I had a troublesome dream. I dreamt that I was sleeping in that very same ICU call room when the nurses called me to a code. I dreamt that I had fallen back to sleep after they called me... every house officer's nightmare.

When I awakened from the dream, I was, of course, in the ICU call room and I actually believed that the dream was reality.

I rushed out to the nursing station and was amazed to see the nurses sitting calmly, writing in their charts. I asked where the code was. I must have been so agitated, because they burst out into laughter. I guess I wasn't the only sleep-deprived intern to have that dream.

THE BRAVE COUPLE

In the ICU, sad experiences greatly outnumbered the funny ones. When patients are close to your own age, their illness has more of an emotional impact on you beyond the usual patient-doctor relationship. Sometimes you identify with them and then you share their suffering more than you should.

A thirty-year-old woman was transferred from the oncology floor to manage the multiple organ complications of her lymphoma and her most recent attempt to treat it with chemotherapy. We knew she was dying and so did she... and so did her husband, eventually.

She was not a typical ICU patient because she was a "no-code." In other words, she did not want to be resuscitated. There were no private rooms available on the oncology service, but we had a quiet room available in the ICU. She needed a peaceful place to die.

We'll call her Angela. She was a pretty girl with a couple of small children and a husband who adored her. Her lymphoma was unresponsive to treatment, and she lay in our bed with bruises from her multiple IVs and blood tests. Those were her battle scars from fighting the good fight, but she was losing. Her husband of about the same age was constantly at her bedside. We'll call him Tony. Whenever I had the time, I would go over and talk to them.

There is a phenomenon in medicine where dying patients aren't visited as frequently by doctors and medical students. Certainly, they make rounds and take care of them, but the social visits drop off. Social visits occur throughout the day when we are passing a patient's room. We would usually drop in just to say hi or to chat a bit. These face-to-face contacts are beneficial for both parties.

When we walk past the room of someone who is dying, however, we take it as a failure on our part. We don't like to be reminded of our failures. Although it is not our intention, these people get less social contact with us. It's a human phenomenon, and doctors are all too human, as I hope you will glean from this book. To this day, I try to be aware of this feeling and I try to compensate for it.

My goal was to keep Angela as comfortable as possible and not let her or her husband feel alone in the cold, clinical intensive care unit. One of the ICU nurses had recently been treated for leukemia and was in remission, so I think she had a special interest in Angela as well. We both spent a lot of time with them.

When I was not in the middle of crises or the never-ending teaching rounds, Tony and I would go to the ICU waiting room and drink coffee. He told me many times that Angela was his whole life, and how their little kids had no idea of how sick Mommy was. He said that he told them she was in the hospital. They were staying with Angela's parents, who knew she was dying. They also took turns visiting.

Tony and I talked about many things; I tried to get his mind off the situation at hand, even if only for a few minutes of reprieve. He had taken time off from his job so he could be with Angela. He had brought the kids in to see her earlier that day. Angela knew this was last time she would ever see them. As we watched from the nursing station, there was not a dry eye.

In the next couple of days, Angela developed pneumonia and she asked that it not be treated. The infection advanced rapidly in her immune-suppressed state, and soon she was unconscious with irregular breathing.

Aside from the busy ICU and all the crises, this took a toll on me. Angela and her husband had been brave about her facing her death and his having to face life without the love of his life. I admired their courage as they broke my heart.

He held her as she died. The nurses and I watched from a distance. I still can't get that image out of my mind. When the alarm on her heart monitor sounded, we turned it off. From the nursing monitor, I watched her heart slow down to the occasional dying-heart beat, and then it stopped completely. I had seen a lot of death in my time, but this was the first time I had witnessed it on a monitor screen.

I looked up and saw that Tony was still hugging his wife. We left him there until it looked like he was ready to let go. I led him away from his wife's body as the nurses went in to prepare her for the morgue.

I walked with Tony out to the waiting room so he could tell their parents. I sat with them for a while and then went back into the ICU.

When I talk about different experiences molding a young doctor, this was one of them. I shall never forget these two people. I confess that I became tearful as I wrote this section of the book.

ANGEL WINGS

The rotation schedule was quite humane about how long we were exposed to the emotional intensity of the ICU. I'm sure it wasn't intentional, but we certainly appreciated only spending a month at a time in it.

Just as the house-staff becomes jaded by being around so much death, so did the nurses. The main difference between the nurses in the ER versus the ICU was that the ER nurses were cynical, while the ICU nurses had a strong sense of humanity that bordered on the metaphysical, if not downright superstitious.

I had just finished placing a subclavian catheter into one of my patients, and one of the older nurses was helping me tape it into place. A subclavian catheter placement is a tricky technique by which a large bore needle is placed parallel and under the collarbone so that a tube can be threaded into the large subclavian vein. This allows large volumes of fluid to be given, should the need arise. (Today, we have safer ways to accomplish this.) I was very proud of the fact that I had never caused a complication with this technique. I guess the nurse saw me grinning as I attached the IV line.

"Not bad for an intern."

"Thanks. It's good to hear that from a grizzled old nurse."

That was the way we talked to each other. She was quite a character, and we hit it off quite well. I felt like she was taking me under her wing and showing me the things that we didn't learn in medical school. She had watched many doctors over the years, and she was glad to share her knowledge and little tips.

When we were back at the nursing desk, she said, "The guy in Room 7 felt angel wings this morning. Do you know what that is?"

"Got me. I have a feeling you're going to tell me though, right?"

"It means he's gonna die."

"Why do you say that?"

"Listen, when somebody tells you that they felt a tingling on their cheeks or around their nose, they're gonna die."

"Seriously?"

"Yeah, we call it angel wings. At least, that's what I call it."

She went on to explain to me that when people feel this fluttering sensation on their skin, it's like the flutter of an angel's wings, preparing to take them home.

I wasn't sure if she was joking. Surely, it had to be a physiological or neurological phenomenon. I had never heard of it before. That night, the man died.

Lesson learned: You never know.

THE PRIVATE MEDICINE SERVICE

After having been on three very intense rotations, I welcomed my start on the private medicine service. It was a very different world from the ward services. I was assigned to the Meyer House Pavilion, which had private floors. I mentioned earlier that they had their own chef at one time.

EDWARD NEWMAN MD

One of the most prominent private doctors in Chicago was Dr. Edward Newman, affectionately called Eddie Newman, as if it was a single word. He was also known as Chicago's Doctor to the Stars. Although he treated luminaries such as Jackie Gleason, Jack Benny, Sammy Davis Jr., Bill Cosby, and others, his patients included doormen and waitresses as well as the mayor of Chicago.

What I learned from Dr. Newman was bluntness and accessibility. He told you things the way they were... He was not known to pull punches. He probably invented accessibility, and his patients had his home telephone number. He happened to be an excellent physician, and he was funny as hell. He was a legend among the house-staff and we all respected him. He would come in to see his patients in the middle of the night if they needed him.

I can still picture him flying down the hallways of Meyer House, his long grey coat flying behind him. He was fast, hence his other nickname, Fast Eddie. At that time, the attendings wore long grey coats and we peasants wore white.

One day I was about to walk into a private room and make rounds on one of Dr. Newman's patients... a foreign dignitary no less. The man was saying that he had to get out of the hospital because he had business to take care of. The following is my recollection of what Dr. Newman said to the man. I repeat these words with the utmost respect for Dr. Newman, who knew how to reach his patients. It went something like this:

"You can't leave here, you're sick and we need to find out what's wrong with you. Listen to me, and you'd better believe me. Your wife is going to leave you, your government is going to forget you, and your kids are going to piss on your grave when you're gone."

The man was shocked; apparently, no one had ever talked to him that way before.

Eddie Newman looked at him and said, "As far as I know, I'm the only one who gives a damn about you, so you'd better follow my advice and stay in the damned hospital."

The man stayed. Dr. Newman knew what he was doing.

Lesson learned: Talk to people using terms that will produce the desired response. I miss you, Dr. Newman.

THE DISTILLED WATER

I wasn't used to being around rich people, so being on the private medical service was an eye-opener. They were generally very polite and pleasant to deal with, but they had their quirks.

For example, I was starting to admit a woman who was coming into the hospital for testing. That certainly doesn't happen these days.

I introduced myself to the woman, who owned a nationwide chain of restaurants.

She looked at my black bag, smiled, and asked me, "Do you have any distilled water?"

I responded, "I suppose we do in the pharmacy. Why do you ask?"

"Because that's the only kind of water I drink." She held up her finger, "Hang on a second."

She picked up the bedside telephone and dialed a number, waiting until someone answered.

"Bring me two gallons of my water and a couple of decent pillows. I might be here a couple of days." She hung up.

The rest of my interview and physical examination were uneventful, and by the time I was finished and was packing up my instruments, her Filipino houseboy came rushing into the room, out of breath, carrying two gallon jugs of distilled water and a couple of large satin pillows under his arm.

As I was leaving the room, she graciously told me to mention her name at any of the restaurants in her chain and they would not charge me. I thanked her, but I knew that was a line I would not be crossing.

Lesson learned: Just because a person has quirks doesn't mean that they are bad.

CLOSE THE DOOR!

In those days, the preferred method of exploring for cancers in the lower G.I. tract was the rigid sigmoidoscope. This was also affectionately known as "the silver sword" because of its appearance... and it had a hilt like Excalibur.

The rigid sigmoidoscope was simply a 25cm shiny metal pipe with a tapered end, which was lubricated and inserted through the anus. The patient had to be crouched on all fours and they really had to be convinced that this was a valid test.

Once the tube was inserted all the way, not a comfortable sensation for the awake patient, the tapered end was then pulled back through the hollow tube to allow viewing of the bowel wall. Long swabs could be inserted to wipe the bowel wall clean and allow for better viewing.

One day I was assisting my attending in one of these procedures. The patient was an obese middle-aged man with a suspicion of colon cancer. We brought him into the procedure room that we had on each floor, and helped him into his undignified "doggy style" position.

The nurse was very good about draping him to minimize his embarrassment.

The attending inserted the sigmoidoscope and pulled out the middle portion. A light at the end was showing the details of the colon wall. He motioned me over to take a look.

As I hunched down and squinted through the tube, I could see the pink wall of the bowel. I heard a rumbling in the patient's belly and saw something heading toward the scope. It was something like being in the subway tunnels in Manhattan and watching a big brown train coming at you.

"Shut the door. Shut the door!" My instructor said, as he quickly flipped down the little doorway at our end of the tube.

"That was close," he said.

I was quite thankful that he was so alert. Fortunately, the patient did not have any cancers that we could see. I think the modern colonoscopy technique is a lot better.

SOCIAL ADMISSION AND BREAKING RIBS

When I was quite new to the private service, I got a call from one of the private internists. He was a very fast talker.

"You the intern on call?"

"Yes, I am..."

"I've got an 83-year-old woman coming in. On her way to the floor right now. Sophie Goldberg (fictitious name for privacy reasons). Social admission. Get her tucked in and I'll come by later tonight..."

Before I had a chance to ask what a social admission was, he had hung up.

A few minutes later, the nurses paged me to say that my patient was in her room — a private room — waiting for me. The nursing note didn't have much, just normal vitals and negative responses to the standard nursing questions; no allergies and she was taking a couple of blood pressure meds, vitamins, and a stool softener. There was no chief complaint on the nursing assessment, only the words, HERE FOR TESTING. Again, not what you see these days in hospitals.

When I entered the room, the elderly Mrs. Goldberg smiled and put down the book she was calmly reading.

"Are you the doctor?" She asked me.

I introduced myself and stood at the bedside.

"Mrs. Goldberg, what brings you to the hospital?"

"My son, Irving. He dropped me off on the way to the airport."

"No, I mean, why are you here in the hospital?"

"Why, because my doctor sent me here. He is a wonderful diagnostician, you know."

To this day, I still wince when people use the word *diagnostician*.

All doctors make diagnoses. That's what we do. It's like saying a truck driver is a very good braker.

I was getting nowhere. She seemed to be alert, breathing normally, had good skin color and clear speech, and she was wearing a lot of jewelry.

"Mrs. Goldberg, what illness brings you here... to the hospital? Why did your internist tell you to come here?"

"I don't know. I guess because he wants to run some tests."

Keeping my calm, I decided to look at the bound paper chart that just came up from medical records.

As best I could tell, she had no chronic diseases other than well-controlled hypertension.

I decided to go directly to a detailed review of systems, asking questions about every organ system a person could have. It seemed to take forever because I didn't know where this was going.

She considered each question for a moment, and then gave me an anecdote. For example, when I asked about chest pain she said, "No but my cousin Sadie has it all the time. She was told to stop smoking..."

On it went; I knew that supper was only a dream that had evaporated long ago. I knew my admissions were piling up and the nurses would be bugging me for admitting orders. I was determined to not be rude or seem impatient. I think I pulled it off. Finally, I was finished!

As I was leaving, Mrs. Goldstein thanked me. I smiled and left the room, wondering if there were any crackers or toast in the med room. I was starving and the cafeteria was closed.

My resident, Lennie, was sitting at the nursing station. He said, "So, what have you got there, an LOL in NAD?"

"You got it."

In the medical world, we have abbreviations for everything. An LOL, in those days, meant "little old lady," and NAD means "no acute distress." In pediatrics, we even used the letters GLM for "good lookin' mom."

Lennie said, "Interns hate social admissions. It's part of the deal, so live with it."

"So, what the hell is a social admission?"

Lennie looked at the nurse and they both laughed.

"It's when a family dumps an elderly person off so they can go on vacation alone. The attendings do it out of mercy for family members when Granny or Grandpa is driving them bonkers."

"Okay, so it's like a temporary Brown Bagger situation for people with money."

"Bingo."

As we sat and swapped cynicisms, an aide ran into the nursing station, frantic.

"Code Blue in 314!"

We all ran down the hall and I was relieved to see it was not Mrs. Goldberg as I ran past her room.

We got to the room and a nurse had already pulled up the headboard and was rolling the frail old woman onto it.

Lennie was the senior house officer so he ran the code.

"Messina, start the chest compressions. Sally, one amp bicarb."

So it unrolled. Respiratory therapy was called, Lennie was intubating, and I was doing chest compressions on this frail old lady. For all I knew, she might have also been a social admission. In those days we would begin resuscitation with a thump to the chest before we started compressions. It was called the "precordial thump", presumably to start the heart.

In medicine, there are certain sounds that give cold chills to non-medical people. One of them is the sound of cracking ribs during a cardiac arrest.

The poor lady having the cardiac arrest was old and arthritic, and probably had osteoporosis. I'm not exactly a brute, but to compress her heart properly with my intertwined fingers, I had to press her sternum down a couple of inches. As I did that, I could feel crunching sounds.

The crunching was probably from me breaking the calcified cartilage connecting her ribs to her sternum, but it also could have been ribs. It made quite an impression on me.

I had been to many arrests by then, but never on such an old person, and never had I personally crunched a chest like that. It would not be my last, not by a long shot.

The code went on around me, Lenny calling out meds, pushing me clear as he shocked her with the defibrillator. On it went. The charge nurse was writing down the meds as they were given. An attending, a respiratory therapist, a nursing supervisor, and two wide-eyed medical students were also crammed into the private room.

The drama continued, but she never regained a cardiac rhythm, despite the well-run code.

"What time is it?" Lenny asked the nurse, as he put his hands on mine to stop my compressions.

"8:52."

"Okay. I'm calling it. No response to resuscitation. Time of death, 8:52 PM.

As I walked back to the nursing station, I passed Mrs. Goldberg's room. She looked up from her book and waved, smiling. She was going to have a much better night than I was.

The eight-week private medicine service was interesting, and I learned a lot from private doctors such as Dr. Newman, but I missed the ward service. I missed taking care of people who were really much sicker than the private patients were.

BACK TO THE ER

After another ward medicine rotation for a month, I was back in the ER to fill in for another intern. At this time, however, they were rebuilding the Michael Reese emergency room and we had to work out of several large shipping containers, the kind that fit on large semi trucks. The hospital engineers had bolted or welded them together and cut holes so we could walk between the different chambers and into what was left of the emergency room during the demolition and reconstruction.

The ER was crazy enough as it was before, but now we had to function in shipping containers!

THE CHANGE WILL DO HIM GOOD

Not everyone that came into the emergency room was a genius, as perhaps you've already noted.

A local homeless guy was brought into the emergency room with shortness of breath. He lived in a doorway, and most of his nutrition came from cheap booze such as sweet Muscatel wine or cheap whiskey. He was quite drunk when he came in.

He told me that he suddenly became short of breath a couple of hours ago. He denied any chest pain or any fevers, although certainly his history was probably not very reliable.

I listened to his chest and I could hear no breath sounds on the left side. I immediately put him on oxygen and got a portable chest x-ray.

I snapped the x-ray films up onto the white fluorescent view box and immediately saw something strange. I called my resident over to take a look.

"Coins?" We said almost in unison.

The pulmonary fellow was still in the house so we got him to put a bronchoscope down. He removed three coins from the airway. He told us that one of them had been acting like a butterfly valve, keeping air from getting to the left lung.

When the patient woke up from the short-acting anesthetic agent, I naturally had to ask him how the coins got into his left main stem bronchus.

He told me that he liked to put pennies or nickels in his mouth when he drank hard liquor because it improved the flavor as it passed over the coins. He would usually drink until he passed out, and this last time he must've been so dead drunk that he choked on the coins.

Lesson learned: Change is not always good for us.

THE *SHPOS* AND ANGEL DUST

One day as I was starting my shift in the makeshift ER, I felt the floor rocking up and down as four cops were wrestling in the narrow hallway with a troublesome individual who the nurses were calling a SHPOS. In some settings, this is the acronym for "State Historic Preservation Officer." In the large urban hospital setting, however, it stood for "Subhuman Piece Of Shit." This term was usually reserved for people who threw up on your feet, bit you, or tried to hurt you in some other way. Sometimes we get very insensitive in healthcare, as I warned you earlier.

The cops had managed to wrestle the guy into one of the exam rooms, but he was throwing them all over the place. The guy was huge and muscular. I could feel our flimsy structure shudder as cop or SHPOS bounced off the walls. I ran into the room — perhaps not a brilliant thing to do at the time.

One of the cops saw me and yelled out as he struggled, "This guy is on dust! You'd better do something!"

He was referring to Angel Dust, otherwise known as PCP. It was phencyclidine, a hallucinogenic agent that was popular on the streets at that time. It can produce feelings of great power and dissociation from reality. Liquid PCP is called embalming fluid. When cigarettes are dipped into it they are known as "wets." PCP produced complete craziness as well as amazing strength. That's what was happening in our examining room. The guy was like a raging bull.

A resident ran into the room, shouting, "What the hell is going on in here?" It was a good question. I took the cue from the policeman and asked the nurses to give him a shot of Haldol. As the cops held him down, she tried to inject the tranquilizer into his arm, but he broke free and he flung her across the room... Dose not given, nurse not injured. But she was pissed!

More people piled into the room until our patient was pinned to the table. One of the nurses brought out some leather restraints. These leather cuffs are about four inches wide, padded on the inside, and they are attached with large straps to the gurney or bed rails. With more struggling and shouting, he was finally placed in four-point restraints.

Although the man's arms and legs were held tightly within the restraints, he was screaming up a storm and arching his back, throwing his head from side to side. It seemed like the gurney would flip over. He was apparently terrified at some terrible hallucinations seen only by him. The first nurse, fortunately unhurt from being thrown across the room, was now able to give him the 5 mg of Haldol that I ordered, intramuscular. It was going to take some doing to get an IV into this guy.

The cops brushed themselves off and left, figuring that we had things under control.

We actually did *not* have things under control. The Haldol didn't touch him, and he started thrashing again, this time tearing loose one of the leather straps. I was frankly amazed to see that. I didn't think a human being could tear the thick leather strap, but he did. He literally ripped the strap, which is thicker leather than the belt that holds up my pants.

Everyone dove onto that one arm that was thrashing around, and I told the nurse to give him another 5 mg of Haldol. It slowed him down a little bit but not enough. He looked wildly around the room, which was filled with medical people, but I don't believe he had any idea of where he was or even *who* he was. He started screaming again and trying to break the rest of the leather restraints as we placed a brand-new leather restraint on the free arm.

We needed to knock him out before he broke his own bones from struggling.

I finally got an IV into him, and we sedated him heavily. Gradually, he came under control.

I was amazed at how strong a human being could actually become under certain circumstances. It makes you pay more attention to those stories where a mother rips the door off a car to rescue her baby.

Lesson learned: When dealing with angel dust, don't be stingy with the tranquilizers.

THE HORROR MOVIE

The Michael Reese PR department gave permission to a Hollywood movie crew to shoot some scenes at our hospital for the film, *The Omen*. They shot footage of the hallways and the nurses at work, and they had some well-known actors come into town for some of the filming. Many of my friends were extras in those scenes.

I, of course, was trapped in the emergency room, disappointed because filmmaking has always been one of my loves. There is something very special about being on a set and watching a movie crew at work. Anyway, in the middle of the day, between crises and cups of coffee, an Assistant Whatchamacallit from the production company came in and wanted to talk to me as the doctor on duty.

"I've got my crew out here in the waiting room, and I want you to give everyone B-12 shots."

I looked at him, wondering if someone had put him up to this as a joke. There were many practical jokers in my class.

"Why would you want that?" I asked, playing along.

"To give everybody more energy. I want them to work harder." He said, arrogantly. He could've been the poster child for little man syndrome.

I realized that he was serious, so I explained to him that it was a myth that B-12 injections gave people energy. I told him that I was not going to do it. I explained how inappropriate it would be.

The Assistant Whatchamacallit got furious and demanded to talk to my supervisor. The attending, who was trying to read journals in the back room, was not happy to be disturbed. He responded as I did to the arrogant little fellow and agreed with me: no B-12 shots.

The guy stormed out of the emergency room. The consequence: should you ever see the film *The Omen*, you will notice that I am conspicuously absent from the crowd scenes. It was a good movie anyway.

Lesson learned: Stick to your guns when you know you are right. It's just not a good way to get into the movies.

NO HOT BUTTERED COOKIE DOUGH

There wasn't much privacy in the shipping containers that served as part of the emergency room. We pulled curtains between the sections, but we could easily hear what people in the next bay were saying.

As I was examining an old lady with pneumonia in one bay, I could hear the surgical intern talking to someone next-door. I couldn't help but overhear as the conversation got more interesting.

"Let me get this straight," the intern said in his thick Indian accent. "You inserted spackle into your rectum?"

"That's right, Doctor." The man said, nervously.

Spackle is like plaster, and it's usually applied in the seams between wallboards before sanding and painting. Sometimes it's available in large tubes with a tapered nozzle at the end, similar to construction glue.

The surgical intern was in great control, judging by his voice. "Please tell me sir, why would you do that?"

The patient sounded somewhat impatient as he responded, "Because I ran out of hot buttered cookie dough." The man said it as if it was a perfectly normal substitution.

The doctor coughed nervously and excused himself. I could hear him running down the rickety floor of the shipping container. I excused myself and ran after him.

I caught him at the nursing station in the main ER. "I couldn't help but overhear what you were saying," I said. "What the hell?"

The young doctor was trying very hard to control himself. I can see that he was trying not to break into laughter, and I was trying very hard as well. It was beyond strange.

"The problem is," the surgical intern said, "when I did a rectal exam, my finger hit a very hard object. It seems to have set. It's like plaster that has become hard."

He showed me the x-ray a few minutes later, and indeed, it looked like a casting of the man's lower colon. There was no way they could remove it rectally, so they took him to the operating room to remove a perfect casting of the lower colon and rectum. I wonder if they saved it as a teaching tool for anatomy.

Lesson learned: Keep your cool no matter what. Nothing is too weird for the emergency room.

SKIN POPPERS

Some days in the emergency room were downright disgusting. I don't think a week went by when I didn't have to deal with skin abscesses in skin poppers.

A skin popper is an addict, usually a heroin addict, who had trouble finding veins. Eventually, they start running out of usable veins so they resort to intradermal injections. This is done by pinching an area of skin, usually the smooth part of the forearm, and injecting heroin or speedball into the skin. Speedballing — or power balling — is when a mixture of heroin and cocaine is injected together. This gives a tremendous rush of euphoria, but sometimes the stimulant effect of the cocaine wears off before the respiratory suppressing effects of the heroin, and the person dies. They stop breathing.

The ones who didn't die often became infected and ended up in our emergency room. Perhaps it was because they didn't observe sterile technique because they didn't go to nursing school.

Typically, a skin popper would show up with an extremely painful abscess of the forearm. There usually were scars from other abscesses in the past. The abscess could be as large as a golf ball with the skin stretched tightly over it. The treatment of choice for any abscess is to drain it. It turned out to be simpler than I thought.

I'll never forget my first skin popper from when I was a medical student. He was a kid, about 19 years old, who was perspiring, moaning, and holding his arm when I walked into the room. I looked at the enormous abscess, bulging from the skin of his forearm, and I knew it was full of pus under pressure, causing the pain. The usual procedure was to take a pointed scalpel blade and simply pop the abscess.

I had asked my intern for some help on how to anesthetize the skin before I stabbed it with the scalpel blade. He motioned for me to follow him.

We walked into the room; he nodded at the patient and reached for a bottle of ethyl chloride. This is the type of solution that sprays from the end of a brown glass bottle. It is commonly is used to freeze the skin because it evaporates so quickly.

He inverted the bottle and began to spray the top of the abscess. Gradually the entire surface of the abscess turned white, like the snowcap on a mountain. It was frozen. He then took the scalpel blade, without using the handle, and pierced the abscess as if he was popping a balloon. The patient still screamed. Fortunately, he held some gauze over the abscess because green pus sprayed out. The patient breathed a sigh of relief almost immediately. We irrigated the abscess and packed it with a long, narrow strip of iodine soaked gauze. It must have been 12 feet long. It amazed me that we could pack so much gauze into this abscess cavity. The patient was happy and I became one step smarter.

Lesson learned: Never be afraid to ask for help.

GETTING IT ON THE SIDE

As long as we're being disgusting, I must tell you about another emergency room encounter.

In that era, it was not unusual for surgeons to connect the small intestine or colon to a bag on the outside of the person's belly. These were called ostomy bags, such as ileostomy or colostomy. Sometimes these were permanent openings, sometimes they were temporary, but they were an endless source of embarrassment for the poor patient who uncontrollably empties their bowel into a bag. They were self-conscious of the sudden sound of liquid stool emptying into the bag.

Many ostomy patients became extremely self-conscious and wore a lot of perfume or cologne, because they felt that there might be odors. Although the ostomies were life saving, in most cases they were a burden to the patient.

On one occasion, I was asked to evaluate a patient who had an infected colostomy opening. She was a middle-aged woman from the projects, and the nurses told me that she used to be a hooker before the colon surgery.

When I examined her, I removed the bag that was attached with adhesive around the one-inch diameter opening. I had seen a number of colostomies from my surgical rotation, but this one looked red and angry. The surgical site was well healed, but there appeared to be pus along the edges of the opening. Instead of the nice pink and healthy intestinal tissue that we normally would see, it was red and bleeding. And there was pus...

I went out to get some culture tubes so I could take a sample to send to the laboratory. When I came back into the room, the woman was looking at me sheepishly.

"I can save you a lot of trouble," she said, "my man and I been having sex down there."

It was then that I realized that this was gonorrhea in a most unusual location.

Lesson learned: People never cease to amaze me.

THE BOSSY NURSE ON 6 MAIN REESE

In January of my internship year, I finally completed my emergency room rotation. It was about 2:00 AM because it had been so busy. I was to begin my rotation on the general Internal Medicine floor at 7:00 AM the next morning.

It wasn't worth driving 20 minutes home and then 20 minutes back again, so I elected to stay in the call room designated for the medicine service where I could catch some sleep and a shower before changing back into my white uniform.

By the time I finally figured out who was sleeping in the different cots in the call room, it was about 2:30 AM. What seemed like seconds later, the night had passed and it was morning. I took a shower, then wandered around until I found some food in the kitchen and grabbed a foam cup of hot coffee.

6 Main Reese was on the sixth floor of the building known as Main Reese. Unlike the research, psychiatry, surgery and other pavilions of Michael Reese, many of which catered to private donors with the finer things of life such as private chefs, Main Reese was for people

who had no money and no insurance (before Medicaid was widely available). This was in keeping with the hospital's longstanding policy to be "Open to all people, regardless of creed, nationality, or race." Despite this, Main Reese was a sight to see.

6 Main Reese was a medical floor consisting of a few individual rooms, but mostly a lot of wards, each containing multiple beds. It had been built in 1907 with high vaulted ceilings and drab paint, but there was plenty of room and there were plenty of beds. There were a few registered nurses on the floor and a lot of nurse's aides and orderlies.

It was not unusual to find the aides and orderlies in supply closets or freight elevators, sleeping or mating — or both. This was the frustration of the charge nurse. Because they were in a union, the charge nurse had very little authority over them.

I stumbled into the main nursing area where I was supposed to meet my new resident and a couple of new medical students. It was the start of a new rotation, and I was looking forward to it. As I sat bleary-eyed at one of the tables, not knowing which of the charts would be assigned to me, I spotted a cute, young, blonde nurse who appeared to be extremely bossy.

She was at the other end of the nursing station from me, and she was telling everyone what to do. From her body language, I could see how frustrated she was with the sullen aides and orderlies who were all but ignoring her. She sent them on their way and flew to another area of the nursing station to give bed assignments to another nurse, and then she dashed into the medication room.

Seconds later, she was back out again with a tray of meds. She swooshed over to where I was sitting, and I could hear the crackle of her starched uniform. She was looming over me and I looked up with a smile.

She had a great smile. She stuck out her hand and said, "Hello, my name is Jayne Bailey and I'm the charge nurse. I assume you're the new intern on the service?"

I stood up and gave her my best grin, introducing myself. I told her that I was indeed the new intern and I was waiting for the rest of the crew. She pointed to a little room off the main area and smiled. "They're in there, probably waiting for you." She swooshed away.

Jayne Bailey, RN, took her work very seriously and she was very efficient. Over the next few days, whenever I looked up, she was swooshing by. She worked energetically and always had a smile for everyone. She was more productive than any two nurses.

As most of the male interns had a tendency to do, I asked her out on a date and she said no. I didn't feel too bad since she seemed to be turning down everyone else as well. She seemed like a real keeper, and I wasn't going to give up. I swear to this day that when I first saw her, she was surrounded by a picket fence in my mind's eye.

SICKLE CELL AND THE EXCHANGE TRANSFUSION

A few days later on morning rounds, my resident assigned me the arduous task of doing an exchange transfusion on a grownup. The patient had sickle cell disease and was being prepared for major surgery. The surgeons kept her on our service because of her sickle cell disease. In those days, we had to replace most of their abnormal blood with healthy blood so that they would tolerate the surgery. Nowadays, sickle cell patients benefit from frequent transfusions to protect them from crises.

Sickle cell disease has to be hell on earth, and may well be the result of bad karma from a past life. We recognized the sickle patients by their moans... You see, they were in pain all the time. During "sickle cell crises", the disease causes small blood vessels to close off, causing painful tissue damage.

Sickle cell anemia is caused by abnormal hemoglobin. Normal blood cells are round and flat with a dimple in the middle. Sickle cells have abnormal hemoglobin that causes them to become crescent shaped and stiff. Where normal red blood cells pass flexibly through the small blood vessels, the sickle cells block blood flow, causing damage to many organs.

Early in the life of a sickle cell victim, the spleen is destroyed from this process, and the patient loses the ability to fight off many infections. Almost any organ can be damaged, including bone, where the blood flow is interrupted and painful bone infarcts develop. These areas of dead tissue often become infected.

Michael Reese had one of the largest sickle cell clinics in the country and was run by Dr. Mabel Koshy and Dr. Margaret Telfer. They were available day and night for their "sicklers" and they knew them all individually. These doctors were the reason why those patients lived as long as they did.

Since dark clouds can produce rain and rain produces flowers, the upside of the long and laborious exchange transfusion was that Nurse Jayne Bailey was going to assist me.

The procedure involved placing an intravenous line in the patient, and utilizing a T-connector with a stopcock, I would use a syringe to extract about 50 cc of bad blood from the patient, turn the stopcock, and squirt it into a receptacle. I would then turn the stopcock in the opposite direction, draw 50 cc of "good blood" from a hanging bag, and gently inject it back into the patient. As primitive as this sounds, it was actually quite effective at the time. It took a long time before we could sufficiently dilute the sickle cell blood with enough normal blood to make surgery safer.

Our patient was heavily medicated for her severe pain, and she didn't seem to mind that I was striking up a strategically planned conversation with Jayne. For Jayne, the procedure must have felt as if it took forever. For me it went all too quickly. We had a chance to talk for quite a while.

Jayne told me that she hailed from Grand Rapids, Michigan, and that coming to the south side of Chicago had been a culture shock for her. I honestly had never heard of Grand Rapids, so she held up her right hand, which was the shape of the state of Michigan and showed me.

She told me that she saw her first cockroach when it was zooming out from beneath a bedside table. She screamed, and one of my colleagues, Myron, ran over to her. When he asked her what was wrong, she just pointed. He angrily told her get used to it, and left her standing there, disgusted. She did get used to it; she was tough and determined.

She told me how she had a little studio apartment in the Prairie Shores complex, which was a row of high-rise apartments on the western edge of the Michael Reese campus. Many of the house-staff and nurses lived there. I was foolish enough to live on the North Side.

She told me how she had to adjust to the way the ward patients lived. Many of the older female patients would use chewing tobacco. When she tried to take their morning oral temperatures, they would tell her to hang on while they took a paper cup and drooled out the brown tobacco juice that they had in their mouths all night long. I don't think she ever really got used to that.

We talked about many things that related to the hospital as well as our own lives.

By the end of the transfusion, as we were taking everything apart, I took another shot at asking her out. She accepted. We were married a few months later, and for some crazy reason, we are still together.

Lesson learned: You can't account for some people's taste.

THE WOMEN'S BOARD RESTAURANT AND CHEESE BLINTZES

In the basement of one of the Kaplan Pavilion at Michael Reese was the famous Women's Board Restaurant. This marvelous eatery was run by the Women's Auxiliary Board of Michael Reese Hospital.

The Women's Board had deep origins in Chicago's German Jewish community, which probably explains why you couldn't get better cheese blintzes anywhere in Chicago.

The usual food source of a Michael Reese intern, when not ordering patient trays for themselves in the intensive care units, took place in the hospital cafeteria. It was not elegant, but I don't think any of us ever got sick from it.

In those days, when you were sitting at one of the long tables with your friends and colleagues, you would always eat the most desirable portion of your tray first, even if it was the desert. The reasoning was simple. When you were paged on the overhead loudspeakers for a specific patient floor, you didn't waste time looking for a telephone; you just dumped your tray and ran to the floor.

The explanation was quite basic. The floor nurses knew that our eating time was sacred, so they only paged us if it was an emergency. We knew that if they paged us, it was important. If it was important, you needed to physically go to the floor.

The only exception was when you were selected to take a potential residency candidate to the Women's Board Restaurant. As I mentioned earlier, hundreds of people interviewed for each of the seats in the medicine residency program. If a candidate was considered a good one, Dr. Sherwood would ask one of the interns to take them on a brief tour of the facility, tell them how happy we were, and then treat them — at the department's expense — to a marvelous lunch at the Women's Board Restaurant.

This was only possible when you were on a predictable service, such as being off hours on an ICU or ER rotation, or on an elective. I was a big fan of being a tour guide, as was Dr. Michael Chin. Whenever possible, we would give our names to Dr. Sherwood's secretary, so we were frequently called upon to undergo the severe hardship of showing off our hospital and eating prime rib and cheese blintzes. I'm sure Dr. Sherwood's secretary was on to our game but she kept calling us.

SNAKING A PATIENT IN THE MIDDLE OF THE NIGHT

Late one night (or early one morning depending how you look at it) I was staggering down the halls of 6 Main Reese on my way down to the emergency room where I had designs on some chewy black coffee before I worked up my next two new admissions.

I ran into a fellow intern, Steve Feinstein, who looked as bad as I did.

"Hi Ed," he said. "Where are you heading?"

"Hey, Steve. Oh, I'm heading down to the ER. I got two more hits from Stu down there. What are you up to?"

"Okay, I'll walk with you. I need some coffee."

We started walking. "So, seriously, what are you up to now?"

As we reached the tunnels, he said, "Well, I don't want to wake up my resident, but I need to do a transtracheal aspirate. Have you ever snaked anybody?"

Steve was referring to the technique where you punch a needle through the upper trachea and carefully thread a thin tube down to where the trachea branches into the bronchi. The idea was to squirt some saline down there and then suck back quickly on the syringe as the patient was coughing in order to get pure culture material from the lung itself. Personally, I really liked the word "snaking" because it just sounded cool.

"Well, I did it once with Schwartz breathing down my neck. It wasn't so tough. You just have to be careful that you don't shear off the tube and drop it into a bronchus when you're pulling it back out past the bevel of the needle."

"Well hell, that makes you an expert. How about showing me?"

And so it went, back to the old "See it, do it, teach it."

THE SLOW X-RAY CLERK

We made it down to the ER quickly and drank some of that thick, caffeine-containing syrup that they called coffee. One of the finest aspects of my time at Michael Reese was the camaraderie, which often took place over that thick coffee. As I poured my coffee, one of the ER nurses told me that my two admissions were on the way up to the floor. I had just missed them.

"Hey Steve, remember that really annoying, lazy, slow-moving woman at the x-ray checkout desk?"

"Yeah. I used to hate going down there to get films on my patients. She was slow and mean. Why?"

"Well, have you seen her lately?"

"Nope, I got three medical students on this rotation, so I send them on the film gathering missions. You know, to enhance their educational experience."

I was pouring my second cup of coffee and I baited him, "What you think is wrong with her?"

"Just plain sluggish, I guess."

"Well, I heard that she was admitted to Meyer House for CHF [congestive heart failure]. It turned out that she had extreme hypothyroidism."

We were walking back to the floor by now; Steve paused, saying, "No shit!"

"Yeah, they have her on thyroid replacement and she's like a new person. I was down there the other day to get some films and she was bright and fast... A new person."

"Like a caterpillar turning into a butterfly."

We made it back to the floor, Steve and I had snaked his patient, and I headed back to my floor. Despite all these admissions — seven that night — I still was able to get two hours of sleep before morning rounds.

Lessons learned: Always help your buddies and never underestimate the power of the thyroid.

THE SCALE INCIDENT

In my era, the better teaching hospitals were the most abusive of their house-staff, at least as it related to workload. Interns were required to do a massive amount of scutwork, which is mostly delegated to others in modern times. Scutwork includes drawing blood, wheeling people down to x-ray, and other tasks perhaps not fitting for someone with our education. We would commonly need to draw our own labs, do our own EKGs, squint through the microscope at a patient's urine, and do anything else it took to get the job done.

Although we complained a lot at the time, I honestly believe that this led to a solid work ethic that is critical to being a proper physician. Despite our massive degree of sleep deprivation, looking back, I truly believe that our patients on those wards got the best of care. We were being overseen by marvelous clinicians who had faculty positions at the University of Chicago. We wanted for no technology available at that time. Michael Reese allowed every patient the same access to the best equipment when it came to testing, surgery, and medical care in general, whether they were on welfare or rich.

Amid the hard work and feelings of not being appreciated, the good news was that we were constantly being taught. Michael Reese was a true teaching hospital, and the Internal Medicine residency program was one of the best in the country. The attending physicians knew who we were and truly shared as much as they could with us.

I think the best type of graduate medical education is the type where the resident has a hands-on experience. In addition, I personally have found it far easier to learn from smart people that I respect. Likewise, I think a lot of residency training has to do with surrounding yourself with smart people; we learned a lot from each other.

It's hard to feel particularly elite when you're the one who has to literally carry your patient over to a scale to weigh them. Shirley, one of my fellow interns, was keeping careful watch on her patient's weight because of fluid retention and kidney failure. The nurses were busy, the aides were nowhere to be found, and Shirley needed to move on with her rounds. It was essential to know the patient's weight, so she enlisted one of the medical students to help lift the debilitated, overweight, and demented patient from the bed and to stand him on a bathroom scale. The idea was to balance him just right to get an accurate reading.

It was a big ward and I was on the other side with problems of my own. As I was slipping a needle into the antecubital vein of my patient to do blood cultures for an FUO (fever of unknown origin), I looked up to see Shirley and her student precariously balancing the old man on the scale. Shirley was standing directly behind this unfortunate patient who had his hospital gown open in the back for the entire world to see.

Perhaps it is insensitive of me to admit this, but I couldn't help but burst into laughter when Shirley was caught by a burst of projectile diarrhea from the poor man who was standing there. He probably wasn't even aware that he did it. As I may have mentioned, interns needed to be dressed in whites at all times, and poor Shirley's uniform became mostly brown.

Her scream caught the attention of the nurses who came to her assistance, and poor Shirley literally ran to the showers. I'm sorry, Shirley, if you read this, but it was damned funny.

PICNIC ON THE GRASS

By the end of my two-month rotation on 6 Main Reese, Jayne and I got in the habit of having lunch together. One day I was walking past Jayne's nursing station, and I stopped to say hi. She held up one finger, signaling me to wait a minute. She was helping an old man who was dressed in the official Michael Reese seersucker robe. He was pushing his IV pole and shuffling in his hospital issued slippers. When she got him into his room, she came back, smiling.

"It's a great day for a picnic," she said.

"Yeah, right."

"No, really. Do you have time to eat outside?"

"Yeah, I have till 1 o'clock attending rounds."

We agreed to meet on the grassy knoll because I had gotten lucky and had almost an hour break. The stars were well aligned on that particular day.

Behind the tall research building and near the emergency room was a beautiful grassy knoll nestled amidst the many pavilions of Michael Reese. On days when the weather was pleasant and temperate, the house-staff would often go out and sit on the grass to try to contemplate normalcy for at least a brief period of time. Behind the knoll was a small store that sold cold cuts, soft drinks, and other such things for the people who lived in the nearby apartments.

I rushed over to the little store and bought some sandwiches, Cokes, and some potato salad. Jayne was already up on the hill, sitting on a blanket and waving at me.

It wasn't unusual to see couples sitting on the grass, eating picnic lunches for that 20 or 30 minutes of peace that they would have. I have very pleasant memories of those days. The nurses would usually borrow white blankets from the linen closets on their floor and spread them out on the grass to have mini-picnics.

On sunny days, the hillside was dotted with young couples on blankets, commonly an intern or resident and a nurse. In my mind, I have this image of beautiful blue skies, green grass, nurses in their white uniforms, and young doctors in their whites, sitting and talking. Sometimes, we polish up our memories when they are special.

We sat and munched on our sandwiches, enjoying the day. It was also a time for hospital gossip.

Suddenly, I blurted, "Did you hear about the shaman over and Meyer house?"

"The what?"

"The shaman. You know, medicine man? Did you hear about that yet?"

She looked at me as if I was joking. She wasn't yet used to the fact that once in a while, I actually wasn't joking.

"Seriously. I wasn't there at the time, but Doug told me that a family had requested a shaman to visit their family member who was a patient here."

"So, what did the shaman do?" I think she thought she was baiting me.

"Well, according to Doug, it was on one of the wards, and they pulled the curtains around the bed. The nurses said they heard something that sounded like a rattle or a maraca, and the guy was chanting. They smelled something burning so they had to go in and tell him to put out the incense or whatever the hell it was."

"You're serious, then?"

"Serious as a heart attack, I responded. Want some more potato salad?" I smiled at her.

We ate for a while and then she spoke.

"What's the story with your resident who wears the surgical cap all the time? I'm sure he doesn't hang around the operating rooms. He has some scabby looking things on his head. I guess he's trying to cover it up. What's wrong with him?"

I chuckled, "Oh yeah. He was going bald so he had some hair plugs transplanted into his scalp. You know, like people do with their lawns. They drill little holes and put plugs of grass into them so they'll spread. I think he was hoping the same thing would happen with his scalp. I wonder where they get the hair." I pointed to a vulgar area.

She giggled and said, "Poor guy."

"Actually, it's kind of ironic. He's on the renal service and they've been using a new blood pressure drug called minoxidil. It seems to work in severe high blood pressure, but it causes a lot of sodium retention. It's kind of paradoxical."

"So why is that ironic?"

"Well, it seems like it causes excessive hair growth on people when they take the drug. Not a very popular medicine for women."

"Yeah, so?"

"Well, I was thinking that maybe they should rub the minoxidil on his head so he'll grow some hair."

We both laughed, not realizing that later the drug would be marketed under the name Rogaine and sold as a hair growth solution.

Although we probably only ate outside a few times, and probably less than a half an hour at a time, it lives in my memory as a time of great piece and contentment. When one considers the things that took place within those hospital walls — the suffering that we witnessed and the frustration at not being able to help everyone — you can understand why these idyllic moments of peace were so important.

A few years later, that beautiful knoll became a parking structure and after that, a pile of rubble.

THE DRUNKEN COUPLE

It was about 2:00 AM, and I was writing one of my last notes on the multiple admissions I had so far that night on call. My resident, Nancy, came up to me and said that we had two hits in the emergency room. She didn't look too pleased, perhaps more displeased than the usual bad news that we would usually get at that time of night. That meant we'd be up the rest of the night.

"You're gonna love this. If we weren't on the receiving end, you'd probably think it was just plain funny. I thought the ER was playing a joke, but it turned out they were really serious."

As we were heading down the elevator and through the tunnel to the ER, she filled me in on the details.

"Apparently these two nasty-looking old people were shacking up and getting seriously drunk. They didn't get out of bed for a few days. Sometimes it's hard to tell drunk from demented, but they probably were both."

"Two days? How is that even possible?"

"Apparently, they paid a cabbie to come by and bring booze and food from time to time. I'm guessing the guy ripped them off each time because they were so out of it."

"So, have you been down there yet?"

Nancy rolled her eyes. "Oh, yes. Like I said, you're gonna love this. You see, they never got out of bed.

They pissed and crapped in the bed, they were so drunk. I shudder to think how their excrescences mingled in the bed sheets. Perhaps they considered it romantic."

"Come on, Nancy. Are you kidding me?"

"No kidding. I couldn't make up something like this."

"So, why are they here in the hospital?"

"Well, I guess the cabbie finally got an attack of conscience. He noticed that the old guy wasn't able to talk, and it wasn't because he was drunk. The old lady looked really sick. So, he called for an ambulance."

By then, we reached the ER. The nurses in their characteristic way were holding their noses and pointing to a couple of the bays on the far end of the ER. I knew that this was not going to be good.

The stench was quite overwhelming. Feces are one thing, but accumulated layers of stale feces mixed with urine and who knows what else are even worse. Lucy pointed to the old man. "Let's start with this one, future neurologist. Here's a good taste of neurology for you."

I went over to the old man and quickly discovered that he was unable to talk and his right side was completely paralyzed. He obviously had had a left cerebral stroke. He was awake enough to know where he was, and he looked very frightened. He frantically tried to talk. He smelled awful. He had no old hospital records and he couldn't talk, so the best I could do was try to ask his bedmate what had happened.

I walked over to the old woman's gurney. She was able to talk, but she didn't make much sense. She was coughing up a lot of discolored sputum and she had a high fever. I stepped out of the area while the technicians took a portable chest x-ray, and then went back in. She also stank pretty badly, needless to say.

The old woman told me between breaths that she and her boyfriend decided to do their drinking in bed. Nancy found her chart and told me that this woman was a chronic alcoholic with end-stage liver disease, as evidenced by her large belly full of fluid. About that time, the cabbie showed up in the emergency room and the nurses showed him back.

He told us that these two people had a tendency to go to bed and just drink. I tried to suppress the extremely unpleasant mental image of them having sex. He said that he they would order pizza from a local place, and they would call him to make a run to the local liquor store a couple of times per day. He said they tipped him pretty well, although I'm sure they had no idea how much they were tipping.

The x-ray came back and the woman had a severe pneumonia, no surprise. By the dark yellow nicotine stains between her fingers, I knew she was obviously a heavy smoker, and that didn't help a bit.

As I was writing my notes on these two unfortunate people, I couldn't help but think about what their lives had to have been like. Where did the roads of life take them so that the two of them could find each other at the bottom of society's scrapheap? Again, as I get corny, I have to realize that these two people were once small children, possibly beloved by their parents... or possibly abused by them.

We admitted both of them to the Ward service. The woman had a resistant strain of pneumonia, and eventually was sent to the ICU where she died a couple of days later. The man survived and eventually was sent out to a nursing home. Neither of them had any family.

Lesson learned: Never get like that.

BLOOD IN THE SNOW

Michael Reese Hospital was an interesting place because of its location. A good amount of violence actually took place within a few hundred feet of the emergency room. Fights would break out and muggings would happen. It didn't seem to matter whether it was day or night.

It was not uncommon for me to see spent 9 mm cartridges in the snow on my way to work. In those days, the police were using .38 caliber revolvers; these were obviously from an automatic pistol. For quite a while, the bad guys were outgunning the cops.

One morning when I didn't have to be on the floor until 8 AM, I was walking across the parking lot from Prairie Shores on the west side of the campus. Jayne had passed this way about an hour earlier for her 7AM shift. It looked like there was blood in the snow, and it looked like someone had been dragged toward the sidewalk, maybe into a car at the curb, because the blood trail stopped right there.

I saw no one in the area, so I started running to Main Reese and I flew up the stairs to 6 East. I was out of breath by the time I got to the nursing station, and I was relieved to see Jayne standing there. She was looking at me with a puzzled expression.

Later that day, I learned that a nurse had been stabbed on the way to work as she was hurrying from Prairie Shores to start her 7 AM shift. It wasn't a nurse that I knew. They found her alive on the other side of campus, but they never caught the guy who stabbed her.

THE COPS AND MICHAEL REESE

I was driving in to work early one morning, heading south on Lakeshore Drive, or LSD as we called it. I was late and speeding to make up time. As I was passing McCormick Place, I heard sirens and saw lights.

"Busted," I said to myself, along with some other choice words.

I pulled over and waited. The cop sat in his car for a moment, figuring I was in a hurry, so naturally he would stress me out for a while and have me wait.

Finally, from my rearview mirror, I saw him walking slowly toward my car, carrying his ticket book, his hand on his revolver.

He looked into my window.

"Going a little fast, there. Where's the fire?"

As I was politely telling him there was no fire, he spotted my hospital ID badge and saw that I was dressed in my whites.

"You a doctor at Reese?" He asked.

I nodded, taking off my badge and handing it to him, along with my license and registration.

He smiled and handed me back my badge. "Heading to work, are you?"

I told him that I was.

"Well, Doc. I'll never give a ticket to a Michael Reese doctor. You never know; one of these days I might be lying on one of your stretchers looking up at you."

He handed my stuff back to me. "Listen, I'm not going to give you a ticket, but please take it easy next time."

I thanked him and started back up, smiling to myself. I guess there were some benefits after all.

Lesson learned: It pays to work at a hospital that had the police contract; we took good care of each other.

BIRTHDAY CANDLES

Following one of the nights when I actually got to sleep at home, I came in the next morning to see one of my colleagues madly scribbling in his chart, grumbling. We'll call him Sid. He was on call the night before. In addition to being tired, he was downright angry.

"Sid, what's up?"

"The surgeons dumped on us again."

"What you mean?" I asked.

"They admitted this guy who supposedly had urinary retention. That sounds like urology, right?"

I nodded. "Yeah, so, why did they send him here?"

"The surgical resident put in a Foley catheter and said that the guy didn't have a surgical problem. Bullshit."

"So what's the plan?"

"This is where it gets weird. We did an IVP last night."

An IVP is an intravenous pyelogram, a test where contrast dye is put in the veins, which is then filtered by the kidney. It outlines the structures of the kidney and its collecting system, including the ureters and down to the bladder.

Sid took me into the next room to show me the IVP films.

"Radiology hasn't seen these yet; look at this!"

He pointed to the bladder. It looked like there were some tubular structures in the bladder. I looked puzzled.

"Those are birthday candles... wax." He almost shouted. "How the hell is this Internal Medicine?"

It seemed that the man had taken some candles, the kind of skinny candles you find on a birthday cake, and he inserted them into his urethra. He pushed a good number of them up his urethra until they started to accumulate in his bladder.

"Apparently, when we were putting the catheter in, there was a lot of resistance, and then things got easy. We must've pushed the final candle into the bladder. He didn't seem to mind it; in fact, he actually smiled as we were doing this. Weird guy. He probably enjoyed it. Yuck!"

I was amazed, "So, how do you propose that they be removed?"

"I'm waiting until the attending gets here, and then he could fight with the urologist about getting the guy operated on. Then we'll call psych."

Lesson learned: There is no such thing as too weird.

THE RENAL SERVICE

The renal service of Michael Reese dealt with disorders of the kidney. The service was run by Dr. Frederic Coe, a great physician and a great teacher.

When the house-staff was presenting a case to him, he would stop us before we told him the blood test results. He would commonly interrupt us and say things like, "Wait! Let me tell *you* what the sodium had to be."

On rounds, he commonly had pearls to share with us. In medicine, a pearl was a tidbit of knowledge that was smart, obscure, and could serve you in the future.

For example, we were doing a consult on a surgical patient whose surgery had been canceled because the surgeons were worried about the low serum potassium level. The patient was a 35-year-old obese woman. The senior medical student presented the case and offered a somewhat inflated explanation as to why the potassium was low.

Dr. Coe listened politely to the student's theory, nodding his head. When we went into the patient's room, he introduced himself to the patient and asked a simple question.

"Do you like licorice?"

The patient said something like, "I love it! How did you know?"

"Just a lucky guess. By the way, how much licorice do you eat?"

"I don't know... I go through a few boxes of Good & Plenty every day."

We followed Dr. Coe out into the hallway.

"How did you know she ate licorice?" The medical student asked.

Dr. Coe responded, "Pseudo-primary aldosteronism can be caused by licorice ingestion. It only takes a few weeks and if, God forbid, the patient is on cardiac medicines, it could produce a very dangerous arrhythmia."

I was very impressed. Many years later, this pearl came in very handy in my private practice.

THE JUNKIE SHUNT

When my resident Marty and I were called to the ER to see one of our chronic kidney patients, one of the nurses pulled us aside.

"He's in Room 4, hemodialysis patient."

Marty asked, "Okay, so, why's he here?"

"He was sent over from the dialysis unit. They refused to hook him up..."

"Why the hell not?"

"You'll see. This guy is a piece of work. Wait till the surgeons see him. They're gonna be so pissed..."

We went into the room. The man recognized Marty.

"Hey, Doc."

"Hey, Lamont. What's going on? Why are you here?"

"The chick in the dialysis unit kicked me out."

Lamont was a man with chronic renal failure caused by his drug addictions. In other words, his kidneys barely worked, so he needed hemodialysis. This is done by attaching an artificial kidney to a specially prepared blood vessel in his arm, called a vascular shunt. When the large needle is stuck into the shunt, his blood goes through a tube and is literally passed through a filtration system, and then returned to his body. He was supposed to go to a dialysis center a few times per week. However, there was a problem with his shunt.

One of the most preciously guarded parts of a dialysis patient's body is the shunt in their arm. It's literally their lifeline. The dialysis shunt was surgically placed in Lamont's forearm by a vascular surgeon by attaching an artery directly to a vein. Normally blood goes from artery to capillaries, and then to the veins, this is a shortcut.

The shunt produced very rapid blood flow, and if you put your hand over these bulging vessels in a shunt patient's forearm, you would feel warmth and a strong humming sensation as the blood sped through. This is where the dialysis machine would be connected so the blood would flow quickly to the dialysis machine and come back into his circulation again.

Marty pulled back Lamont's sleeve.

"Ain't no pulse there, Doc."

We looked at the shunt site. It was swollen and there was pus oozing from it. Marty looked at me and pointed to the needle tracks along the bulging shunt vessel.

"Jeeze, Lamont. Are you still shooting up? In your shunt, for God's sake!"

Lamont didn't answer. He was a hard-core addict and small-time pusher who got an even better rush when he injected the heroin directly into the arterial circulation... better than an IV fix.

Marty listened to Lamont's heart and his eyebrows went up as he was looking at me. He motioned for me to listen to the man's heart.

My time on Dr. G's cardiac service had not been wasted. "Murmur, aortic regurgitation," I said with confidence.

"Bingo. Okay, Lamont has to come on in. You can start doing your H&P now; I'll get the ball rolling with the nurses."

When I heard it was a heart murmur that was probably caused by an infection of the aortic heart valve (and possibly lethal), I grabbed Lamont's thick paper chart and started going through it. It took me an hour, plus the time to take an updated history and do a thorough general examination.

As I was sitting at the nursing desk writing my orders, I saw the surgical resident going into Lamont's cubicle. I could hear him swearing from where I sat. Creating a viable fistula or shunt for dialysis takes a lot of surgical effort; there are only so many available sites.

The surgeons took Lamont to the OR directly from the emergency room, and I heard that they had no success in rescuing the shunt. It was completely infected and they wouldn't operate on the other arm until the infection was cleared up.

Lamont was ultimately admitted to our service. We kept him on antibiotics. His lab tests were quite abnormal since he hadn't been to his last dialysis appointment. We were planning on doing peritoneal dialysis, which I describe later.

When I came in the next morning, Lamont was gone. He apparently had signed out of the hospital AMA (against medical advice). Because he was also a pusher, we figured that he was afraid of losing his customers and his supplier. I never saw Lamont again. Perhaps the emergency room intern pronounced him dead on the Meat Wagon a few days later.

THE ENEMA THERAPIST AND KIDNEY FAILURE

The renal service admitted patients with any dysfunction of the kidneys, especially acute and chronic renal failure. In addition to the more modern hemodialysis, many of our patients were still undergoing peritoneal dialysis.

Peritoneal dialysis is a technique where large amounts of fluid are circulated through the space around the intestines. This is done through an artificial hole in the patient's belly, to which a type of catheter is attached. It's time-consuming and quite unpleasant, but it does preserve life.

Peritoneal dialysis patients would commonly get into trouble because they were often noncompliant and got infections in their belly.

One of our regulars, Sammy, had been lost to follow-up for a couple of weeks. He showed up in the emergency room extremely uremic. This means that he was not getting the toxins removed from his bloodstream because his kidneys had stopped working. When he got to the ER, he was becoming less responsive and very sick. He had not been using his peritoneal dialysis, mumbling to the nurses that he hated it.

What we didn't understand was how he had lived this long without being dialyzed. A couple of days after admission when he was starting to make more sense, we asked him where he had been all that time. Surely, we figured, he had to been dialyzed somewhere because he could never have lived that long without it.

Apparently, Sammy had been seeing an "enema therapist" somewhere on the south side. Apparently this person would do high colonic cleansing enemas for hours at a time. She claimed they would help cleanse the toxins out of his body because his kidneys couldn't do it. He went to her daily for a couple of weeks until he ran out of money and came back to us.

We never did understand exactly what that enema therapist was doing, but I often wonder whether the constant presence of fluid in his colon was somehow serving as dialysis.

LIKE A HOLE IN THE HEAD

I was in the process of doing a physical on one of the kidney patients who had been admitted dozens of times before. This was a man who was generally noncompliant and often got into trouble because he didn't use his peritoneal dialysis properly. His previous admitting notes all looked to be almost identical. He always had the same admitting diagnosis — chronic renal failure — and he always got into trouble after he was discharged. It's amazing that he continued to survive.

Perhaps because I was going to begin a Neurology residency soon, I spent more time with his neurologic exam, which included palpating his skull. I was surprised to feel an indentation in his skull located on the right side. It was an actual indentation, like someone pressed his or her thumb into a piece of clay. I expected him to jump or complain of pain, but he did nothing.

I asked him, "has anyone ever operated on your head?"

"Nope."

I looked at the many scars on his forehead and scalp where he no doubt had stitches in the past from various scuffles in the neighborhood.

"Ever had a skull x-ray? You know, an x-ray of your head?"

"Yeah. About five years ago. Nothing was broken."

I re-examined him and saw no scars around the indentation to suggest a previous burr hole. I sent him for a skull x-ray when I finished my examination.

Later in the day during x-ray rounds, I looked at his skull films. Indeed, on the right side of his cranium there was a hole in the bone that was the size of a quarter. It had irregular edges and some of the edges were denser than others. It did not look like a surgical procedure had been done.

I had the neurosurgeons come by and take a look at him, and they biopsied the bone. It turned out to be a tumor of the bone itself.

Lesson learned: There are no shortcuts in medicine. Always do a thorough exam.

THE TAXI DRIVER

In the midst of my internship when I had time between ER shifts, I would drive across town to Rush Medical Center where Dr. Klawans had relocated. As I mentioned earlier, he was sponsoring a research project I had designed. At the time, I believed that I was developing a new way to diagnose Parkinson's disease by looking at patient autonomic reactions to auditory stimuli.

Whenever I had time, I would rush over and work on the project. On one of those days, I was driving past Rush and I had to stop at a traffic light on Harrison Street almost in front of Cook County Hospital.

There was a red light, and I stopped behind a Yellow Cab. I put my little Mustang II into neutral. I kept my foot on the brake, but I must have dozed off. It was probably only a matter of seconds because the light still hadn't changed. My foot must have slipped off the brake, and the car rolled forward a few inches, tapping the solid steel I-beam, which served as the taxi's rear bumper. It woke me up and the car was still in neutral. My brain said the obligatory, "Oh Shit," that accompanies most traffic accidents.

I pulled up my emergency brake and I jumped out of the car to see the other driver. If you have ever seen a Mustang II, you would know that it was a very lightweight car that was somewhat fragile with a lot of plastic in the front. I'm sure it didn't even budge the taxicab.

I walked over to where the cabbie was sitting, looking somewhat annoyed.

"Are you okay?" I asked.

The cabbie looked at me, noticing my white uniform and hospital ID badge.

His hand went to the back of his neck and he asked, "You a doctor?"

"Yes, I am." I pointed across the street to Cook County Hospital. "Come on, let's get you checked out."

"Uh Uh." He was now rubbing his neck with both hands. "I can't move. I'm gonna call my supervisor. I don't think I can finish my shift." He looked at my badge and wrote down my name on his pad.

The light had changed and people behind us were honking. A policeman who was standing in front of the hospital walked over to the scene and waved the traffic around us.

He walked over and asked, "What's going on here?"

The cabbie told him that he was injured because I smashed into the back of his cab. The cop walked over to where my car had touched his bumper. There was not a scratch on my car, despite the massive steel bumper of the taxicab.

The cop pulled me aside and said, "That guy is trying to scam you. I'm not even going to make out an accident report because this is nothing. You can just take off; I'll deal with him."

I got back in my car and drove back to Michael Reese because my ER shift was about to start.

About three days later, one of the emergency room nurses handed me an envelope. It had arrived at the administration offices, and they found out where I was rotating and sent it to the ER.

The envelope contained a scrawled, almost illiterate, note written on paper that appeared to be torn from a spiral notebook. It was from the cab driver, and it stated that he was injured to such an extent that he was unable to work "ever again." He told me that I would hear from his lawyer.

I knew it was a scam, so I sent it to my insurance agent who told me not to worry about it. It still made me nervous, but over the coming months, I even forgot about it.

Four years later when I had first gone into private practice, I got a letter from my insurance company. They said that the cabbie was suing me for one million dollars because he had been unable to work since the accident.

They also mentioned that it was certainly a fraudulent claim, and they had a special firm that dealt with the sleazy law firm that represented this man. They suggested that he was probably tracking my career to find out when I was actually making a living. They said not to worry, but I worried. The joke was on him because I had a negative net worth.

About a year later, State Farm wrote me another letter saying that they had settled for only $500 and the case was closed.

Lesson learned: When you're a doctor, you are a great target for scam artists. This was a glimpse of the things to come.

MY LAST SERVICE

My last clinical rotation was inpatient oncology in the Baumgarten Pavilion. I had saved my two-week vacation for the end of my internship so I could move to St. Louis and get settled before I started my neurology residency at Washington University and Barnes Hospital.

Inpatient oncology was a tough service. It was the cancer floor, and everyone on the service was being evaluated or treated for cancer. These patients were getting chemotherapy and/or radiation therapy and were immunologically compromised by the medicines we used at the time. They could get infections at the drop of a hat.

People might look stable by day, but by night spike high fevers. Sometimes the fevers were from the chemotherapy, and sometimes it was because of infection. These patients were fighting to beat cancer, so we fought hard so they would not succumb to infections.

A typical night of call involved getting the inevitable nursing calls for fever spikes. When this happened, we would look for any possible cause of infection in the lungs, urine, skin... anywhere. We routinely did blood cultures to look for sepsis. In those days, the intern or medical student would personally perform the ritual of taking blood for blood cultures under the most sterile conditions to avoid contaminating the specimens.

Needless to say, night call was no picnic, and sleep was unusual on our call nights. We were on call every third night.

It was a heartbreaking service because patients spent a lot of time in hospital (unlike today) and we became attached to our patients. It was awful to get a call that your patient was in trouble. Sometimes it was infection; sometimes it was bleeding because their platelet counts had dropped. Pain was another issue, and we went out of our way to be humane. Cancer pain is no walk in the park.

THE RED DEATH

I used to wear a goofy, wide tie to work every day. It was almost in style at the time. There were red spots on the tie that looked like part of the corny picture of two people on the railing of a boat, taking a midnight cruise. The red spots were not part of the original tie but were spots from sprayed doxorubicin (Adriamycin), which happened sometimes when I would draw it into a syringe. It would spatter.

Because the medication was so tricky to administer, the doctor had to give it... slowly injecting it into a vein. We had to be very careful because if it leaked out into surrounding tissue, it could destroy skin or muscle.

The nickname that the house-staff had for Adriamycin was The Red Death because it was so powerful and so dangerous. People would have reddish urine for a couple of days after each dose.

I think the reason I kept wearing the same tie, other than the fact that I have no fashion sense, is because it reminded me of the medication and the need to be ever vigilant.

When we used that medication, we watched people like a hawk and checked their labs frequently.

THE BROKEN NOSE

It worked out well that the end of the year's festivities for the house-staff occurred while I was on the oncology service. I think that the oncology service was the most emotionally draining rotation of my career, including the years to come. I needed the few hours of comic relief.

One of the festivities was the annual softball game between the house-staff and the attending staff. I was lucky not to be on call the day of the event, which was held in a field on the far side of the medical center.

Actually, the very first softball game, ever, was played in 1887 at the Farragut Boat Club, which was on Michael Reese property at the time, so we were carrying out an old tradition.

Our teams were something to behold. On one team were the attendings, older than the house-staff and often not realizing it. The house-staff were younger but we were usually not known for our athletic prowess. We also had the disadvantage of being dangerously sleep deprived. I think that the women on our team were more likely to have been athletes in high school than we were.

To give you an idea of how pathetic our teams were, I was playing center field. Although I always liked playing baseball as a kid, I was never the kid that was picked first when we were choosing sides.

At any rate, the game was off to a great start, nurses and other house-staff and attendings' families were cheering everyone on. People not on call were drinking beer from coolers... including some of the players. It was interesting to see coworkers in clothing that was not whites or scrubs. There's something downright democratic about a bunch of young and old doctors dressed in shorts and jeans and T-shirts. Some of us even had baseball caps.

Before long, there was an injury. A well-known oncology attending was hit square in the face with a pop fly. We had to interrupt the game to give him first aid, and a few of us took him across the field to the ER. As I recall, he had a broken nose.

The game continued and the rest of the injuries were limited to strains and sprains.

THE FANGS AND THE GIRL WITH CANCER

It seemed like the oncology service consisted mainly of me taking blood out of people's veins or injecting things into their veins. Patients sometimes called me The Vampire when I walked into their rooms.

The nurses on the oncology floor were an interesting lot. Like many people dealing with cancer, they had a very optimistic perspective, even when it was not realistic. They became very attached to their patients, many of whom were readmitted on multiple occasions over a period of a year or more, if they lived that long. These people were fighters.

I had one senior medical student assigned to me on that service, a student who at best could be described as flat. We'll call him Mitchell.

One morning after work rounds, one of the nurses came up to me, frowning.

"This medical student of yours is a real dud. I think he makes people more depressed than when they started out. You need to talk to him."

Mitchell wore a bowtie and never smiled. He looked at me like I was speaking a foreign language whenever I cracked a joke. By now, you need to realize that a sense of humor is part of our survival in medicine. Sometimes our humor gets rather dark, but it still serves its purpose. Some people call it gallows humor.

As an intern almost finished with training, it was my job to try to impart as much knowledge as possible to my medical student. Mitchell was bright and he read a lot. He was very up-to-date on the types of cancer we were treating, and he had an in-depth knowledge of the pharmacology of the drugs we used.

The difference between a senior medical student and an intern is simple. The senior medical student goes home every night and gets to read the latest literature, while the intern stays up all night and does all the actual work. As I said earlier, interns usually hate senior medical students. I remember that feeling when I was a senior medical student, and I must admit, I was a pain in the ass.

What Mitchell did not understand was how to relate to other people. I watched him talk to patients, and it was like watching a robot recite. He was very clinical and matter of fact but never smiled or made the patient feel at ease. After the nurses urging, I decided to take him aside one day.

"Mitch," I said, noting that he didn't like that informality. "You gotta lighten up a little."

"What do you mean?"

"I mean, you need to help these people deal with their fears. They know they're sick... very sick."

"I know. A lot of these people are probably going to die before the year is up."

"Yeah. That's the point. We have to try to make them comfortable as much as we can. It doesn't hurt to get a little bit sociable at times."

"You mean, like tell them jokes or something?"

"Something like that. Here watch this."

He followed me down to a room where a patient was lying quietly. Cindy was a 20-year-old girl with Hodgkin's disease. She was trying to finish out her year at the University of Chicago. She hadn't had any visitors for a couple of days since her family lived on the East Coast. Her friends must have felt uncomfortable around dying people, so they tended not to visit. Even her boyfriend seemed to keep away. She was looking down at all the bruises on her arms from IVs that had gone bad.

As Mitchell and I walked into the room, I reached into the pocket of my white coat and pulled out a pair of plastic vampire fangs... The kind you buy in joke stores for Halloween.

I popped the fangs into my mouth and made a wide vampire smile just as Cindy looked up. She cracked up and started laughing loudly. She even snorted.

I looked over at Mitchell and he looked back at me blankly. I'm certain that he thought I was insane, but after a few seconds, I think he got it. He smiled.

"Cindy," I said. The vampire teeth made my words slurred. I sat on the edge of the bed. "My friend Mitchell and I thought we would come in and give you a hard time. He also goes to U of C.... Med school."

Cindy looked so pale and tired but she lit up and smiled, "Really?"

Her smile melted some of Mitchell's anxiety. Looking back, I think he probably had social anxiety disorder. He actually started to speak.

"Yes. So tell me, what's your major?"

"Biology. I'm applying for grad school; I'm very interested in cellular physiology."

And so it went, a complete conversation ensued. Mitchell learned that we also needed to talk to our patients and make them feel comfortable and not alone. Sadly, Cindy's cancer was not responding to treatment and we didn't have much left to offer her.

Mitchell knew this from reading her chart, but he kept on talking.

I left them to chat as I sadly walked out of the room. I knew Cindy would never get to graduate school. You just never get used to certain types of pain.

Lesson learned: Sometimes you have to get downright silly to bring a medical student out of their shell.

EDDIE'S NEWMAN'S PARTY -- THE END OF A GREAT YEAR

Dr. Eddie Newman, physician to the stars, was a very generous man. To show appreciation to the intern class, he threw a party. It was held at a fancy Chicago restaurant known as Arnie's, a steakhouse where Frank Sinatra was rumored to have eaten whenever he visited Chicago. Eddie Newman made it very clear that the sky was the limit and we could order anything we wanted. We seemed to have the run of the place.

It was a remarkable evening. The interns were all relieved of call and other clinical duties while the residents and attendings covered the floors for the evening and night. We didn't know what kind of mess we would inherit the next morning when we went back, but we didn't care.

It was a formal affair, and he told us to bring dates. There must have been at least 50 of us there. It had been a tough year and Eddie Newman knew that we all deserved a break. The guys were dressed in suits and the girls were dressed to the nines. It was like a glimpse into the future. It was what we all might look like when we finally became practicing doctors and had a place in polite society.

I took Jayne. When I saw her dressed up, I had never seen her look so lovely. We sat with two other interns and their dates, also Michael Reese nurses. It was a medical table, which is not always a good thing.

Inevitably, when young doctors get together at a social gathering, the only thing they can talk about is... medicine.

Conversations sounded like, "Did you see that guy this morning with a white count of 40,000?" Or, "I got 12 admissions last night and one of them walked out before I could even get to him. Brown bagger, I thought... Turned out to be just a SHPOS."

Jayne and I looked at each other and just smiled. In just a couple of days, we would be leaving Chicago for our great adventure in St. Louis.

As I looked around at the room, I remembered how green we all were on that first day and how confident we had become. We went through some very hard times together and learned to trust each other. We stood shoulder to shoulder against massive amounts of work and helped each other whenever we could. When we signed out our patients to the intern on call, we had confidence that they would do a good job. We trusted them with our patients' lives and we were never disappointed.

Some of us, like me, were only spending one year at Reese and moving on to subspecialty training at places like Harvard, Johns Hopkins and Washington University. Others were going to stay for two more years to complete their Internal Medicine training before going into their respective subspecialties. Others would practice straight Internal Medicine.

Although it has been many years since then, Jayne and I still reminisce about the Michael Reese Department of Medicine intern class of 1978. There was no finer collection of doctors anywhere, and I am proud to have been part of this wonderful group. As I said in the beginning of this book, it was my dream to be a Michael Reese intern and it came true. The next dream was to follow.

Two days later, Jayne and I packed up an old U-Haul with books and our few possessions and moved to St. Louis where I was to begin my Neurology residency. The adventures over the next three years would further change me and mold me into a neurologist. The story will continue in the second book of this series.

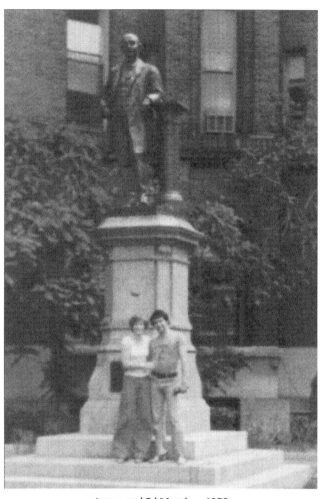

Jayne and Ed Messina, 1978

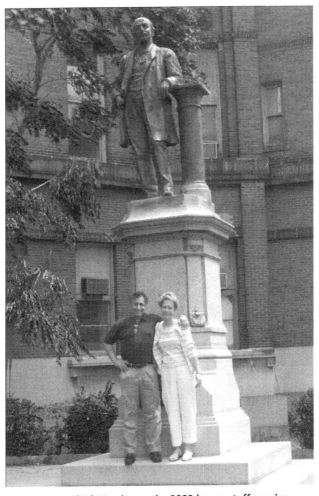

Jayne and Ed Messina at the 2003 house-staff reunion

ABOUT THE AUTHOR

Dr. Edmund Messina was born in Brooklyn, New York, in 1946. A lifelong writer and occasional filmmaker, he lives in Michigan with his wife Jayne, who appears in this book. They continue to work together at the Michigan Headache Clinic in East Lansing, Michigan, a clinic they jointly founded. They have three grown children, Daniel, Jill and Marc.

The Spattered White Coat is the story of Dr. Messina's initiation into the world of medicine. Following his internship at the former Michael Reese Medical Center, he went on to a Neurology residency at Washington University and Barnes Hospital, St. Louis, Missouri.

He is board certified in Neurology by the American Board of Neurology and Psychiatry, is certified in the subspecialty of Headache Medicine by the United Council for Neurologic Subspecialties, and is a Fellow of the American Headache Society. He is Clinical Associate Professor of Medicine in the College of Human Medicine at Michigan State University.

His nonfiction writing also includes multiple scientific and educational projects, including *Evaluation of the Headache Patient in the Computer Age* (Chapter), in *Headache and Migraine: Biology and Management*, Ed. Seymour Diamond MD, Elsevier, 2015.

He wrote and co-directed the documentary, *Life and Migraine* (shown on PBS), and wrote and directed the dramatic feature film, *Lily's Mom*. Released in 2011, the film highlights self-advocacy in health care, and was the recipient of an independent film festival Drama Award and was nominated for Hollywood's Voice Award in 2012 because of its depiction of domestic abuse.

Made in the USA
Lexington, KY
09 October 2016